T0105529

Other books by Frank Burdett

The Rhyme of the Ancient Campaigner.
(A True Story in 270 Rhyming Verses)

The Sons of the Brave.

*Laughing at Yourself About Almost
Anything and Everything.*

Adventures Along the Oregon Trail.

Manuscripts under Revision:
Mountain Man: Man of Stone!
The Prairie Winds Are Crying.
The Indian White Woman.
The Wisdom of Black Crow.
The Purple Tree.

I SURVIVED METASTACISED MELANOMA CANCER!

Hope For Melanoma Sufferers

Frank E. Burdett

BALBOA.
PRESS

A DIVISION OF HAY HOUSE

Punch-Line Publications
2 Lake Street, Varsity Lakes, Gold Coast, Qld.
Email: larfagain23@gmail.com
ISBN 978-0-9807673-2-2

Balboa Press books may be ordered through booksellers or by contacting:

Balboa Press
A Division of Hay House
1663 Liberty Drive
Bloomington, IN 47403
www.balboapress.com.au
1-(877) 407-4847

ISBN: 978-1-4525-0679-1 (sc)
ISBN: 978-1-4525-0685-2 (e)

Printed in the United States of America

Balboa Press rev. date: 09/07/2012

Acknowledgements

I should like to acknowledge the following people who contributed to saving my life!

My dear wife, JEANNE FROST,
who was my caregiver for three years.

VERNON JOHNSTON, Cancer Survivor,
California, USA
whose fine example in having the courage to walk
the steps into the field of alternative treatment—
and survived!

GRAEME ANDERSON,
of Macleay Island, Redland Bay, Queensland,
who gave me such help and encouragement.
Sadly, Graeme passed away in early 2012.

DOMINIQUE FINNEY, BHsc., ND,
of the Sunshine Coast, who was highly instrumental
in helping me fight my cancer.

DON GEARD,
my dear, departed, life-long friend, who gave
me encouragement during my cancer journey.

::

During my personal journey of recovery from stage IV melanoma cancer, I kept remembering that today is the tomorrow I worried about yesterday! Therefore . . . I can easily say: NO MORE WORRIES!

The challenge is to live life to the full or not live life at all, but, to be consumed by not knowing anything, because, to live without experience is no life at all. To hope: is to challenge pain and fear. To try: is to tempt failure. To love: is to risk not being loved in return. However, the greatest failure in life is to risk nothing!

Dedication

This book is dedicated to
CURTIS JOHN MITCHELL
of New York City.

In 2009, Curtis wrote me a wonderful letter of encourage-ment during my early period of stage IV metastacised melanoma cancer. This was after I had initially been informed by the medical profession that I had up to six months to live. I was so impressed with Curtis' letter that I should like to share it with my readers. And, what better location than in a place of dedication. Here, then, is that important missive.

Frank,

Enjoy the experience of Cancer! It can be more fun than folks lead on to; more beautiful in the moment than society can grasp. Find your breath in the moment and you'll be able to observe and be in line with whom you really are from your true place of being. Cancer does not exist with who you really are, nor will it ever affect you there.

I think the hardest part of the journey, such as Cancer, is other people's beliefs. Be aware of them and how they limit you. Some folks move beyond the diagnosis of Medical Doctors when they believe they can.

My prognosis was paralysis and/or death and, either I am still dreaming when I snowboard and hike mountains and kayak and do all the things they said I would never do again, or else, beliefs play a large role in reality and maybe miracles are more in line with them. Breathe deep, Mate!

Curtis John Mitchell,
New York, 2009

Table of Contents

List of Illustrations

A Brief Explanation of Melanoma Cancer

Melanoma is a malignant tumour of melanocytes. These are cells that produce the dark pigment melanin, which is responsible for the colour of skin. Melanomas are not common, however, they are more dangerous and cause the majority of deaths related to skin cancer. The diagnosis is more frequent in women than in men and is particularly common among Caucasians, especially northern Europeans living in sunny climates with high rates of incidence in Australia, New Zealand, North America (especially Texas and Florida) and Latin America. There is a slight decrease in southern Italy and Sicily. This geographic pattern reflects the primary cause, ultraviolet light (UV) exposure, crossed with the degree of skin pigmentation in the population.

Cancer cells thrive in an acidic environment, yet they perish in an alkaline, high pH environment. Although many natural nutritional diets assist cancer patients, including stage IV cancer patients, proven alternative treatments for metastacised melanoma cancer receive almost no favourable publicity. More and more people are learning of the benefits of alternative treatments and I am one who has genuine proof that alternative treatments can be life-saving.

In my own experiences, I found that being diagnosed with metastacised cancer can leave you feeling overwhelmed, scared and alone—totally alone! Therefore, educating yourself is an important step towards control. Also, talking to other people who have had metastacised melanoma cancer can help ease a person's feeling of isolation. That is the main reason why I wrote this book—to offer genuine hope to sufferers of metastacised melanoma cancer. There is hope available to metastacised cancer sufferers within these pages.

Author's Note

Living on an island may sound an idealistic existence. It is, until one is confronted with cancer and the ramifications of that disease, which causes numerous problems that have a stress all of its own. We lived on the greatest secret in Australia (at the time), on Macleay Island in Morton Bay, a marine reserve, fifteen minutes from Redland Bay. My wife, Jeannie, and I lived contentedly on the island for seven years enjoying the colourful birds, the tranquil atmosphere and the overall lifestyle. Jeannie was happy painting her abstract art while I wrote books. One day I suddenly noticed a small lump on the left-hand side of my shoulder near the neck. I mentioned this to Jeannie and we decided I had better get it checked out immediately.

It was Saturday when Jeannie phoned our mainland doctor who instructed us to visit him the following day. He completed his examination, shook his head, and stated that a biopsy needed to be taken. This was arranged for Monday. The biopsy, of course, was diagnosed as positive melanoma cancer.

This was the beginning of a two and a-half year metastacised melanoma cancer journey, which was shared by Jeannie, who was my caregiver throughout this whole period. The journey was not the same journey for Jeannie as it was for me—it was my melanoma cancer, but I was Jeannie's husband and therefore the level of stress was more for her as she never knew what further stress she might have to face.

This story looks at the strengths of our relationship, despite the difficulties of living on an island. It is interesting how we were aware of these difficulties, yet worked through them. Included are the details of how the cancer was treated, both by orthodox treatment and an alternative treatment. My alternative treatment had a special journey all of its own, incorporating several people, all of whom were heroes in their own right. This alternative treatment was later to have a dramatic effect upon the Brisbane oncologists as they were astonished with my CT scan results. They asked me what I had taken and regarded this result as a miracle.

It is a thoughtful, painful and revealing account of the years that Jeannie and I would not want to repeat. This story is educative with a thorough report and a message that brings genuine hope for those who now have seemingly little hope against melanoma cancer.

Introduction

How best am I able to process such an emotional subject as metastacised melanoma cancer, especially when stage IV cancer is recognised by orthodox medicine as being a definite death sentence? I reasoned that many people would have great difficulty in accepting my miracle story—even if such a dramatic description had been expressed by oncologists at a Brisbane hospital! I had a certain degree of difficulty in accepting that I was the main character of this phenomenon!

Miracles are interlaced with certain religious connotations, but, as I am not a practising religious person, I am discombobulated as to how I was chosen to be bestowed with the wonder of a miracle. I could possibly be considered as having a persuasion towards spiritual things, as I had personal experience of spiritual events when I served in Malaya in a military role where I cohabitated with Malayan Aboriginal people, many of whom had not met a white man before! These people were from a remote region of the deep inner jungle regions known as the "Ulu". But I digress!

The only way that I could come to terms with this miracle phenomena was to express it through the written word. Expressive writing has been shown to help people heal—emotionally, mentally and physically. When someone writes their deep thoughts and feelings about traumatic events in their lives—and cancer is certainly a traumatic event—their blood pressure decreases, their heart rates slows, and they produce more lymphocytes, which is a type of white blood cell that boosts the immune system[1].

As an aside, I should like to offer that I had a unique experience, inasmuch that while in Malaya, I was attacked, mauled and carried off into the surrounding jungle by a man-eating tiger whose victims to that date were seven humans. It is a true story and I have the scars to prove it! I survived that experience by maintaining a positive attitude and, therefore, I feel qualified to state I am a true survivor! I have inserted this tiger experience in explanation that I can honestly say . . . "Never give up on hope, or positive thinking!"

Before writing fully about my unique tiger experience I wrote a 270 rhyming verse poem, entitled, The Rhyme of the Ancient Campaigner. This was in the form of self-counselling as I had received no professional counselling at that time and also, as a clarification for my grandchildren as to my reasons for volunteering for military service in Malaya. I wanted to enlighten them as to how I survived such an attack, and other side issues that had devastating effects, not only upon me, but upon my fellow patrol members. I was asked by many people to expand on the episode, which resulted in a successful book, Sons of the Brave. It is now a part of history that not many people are even aware there was a 12-year war in Malaya!

I received an email from a New Zealand soldier who wanted to purchase a copy of Sons of the Brave. I replied that the book had sold out, explaining I had written a revision, but due to hospitalisation, I had put everything to one side as I was not expected to survive this present ordeal. The soldier asked if he could visit me in Queensland to discuss my revised edition, which was now sitting in the drawer of my "office" at home.

Jeannie and I met with Peter Jones and his wife, Bev, for morning tea in Cleveland. It was then that Peter offered to process the revised edition, organising its publication and marketing in New Zealand as he offered the book would be published at a reasonable price. However, the work sold better than initially expected, with a response for a further printing.

During my cancer journey I penned another work that was fortunately well received. Researching and writing helped me relieve the stress along the journey. Following overcoming the trauma of my diagnosis of melanoma cancer, I directed my energy towards exploring melanoma cancer for the purpose of helping other melanoma cancer patients to heal. I thoroughly researched what I considered was important, feeling deeply about each subject. Some people revise their journals and notes and reread them thoroughly. I didn't consider that necessary in order to reap the healing effects. During further research, I discovered many of the early pioneers of cancer treatments, several of whom were courageous in expressing their findings. But, finally, most were ignored and even belittled by orthodox medical professionals. Even as I write, several findings of those early pioneers are being re-examined with excellent results emanating from their source.

Here is just one example: In the 1920s, Johanna Brandt suggested her 100% cure rate using purple grapes (i.e., the Brandt Grape Cure). Her proven treatment was ignored by the medical community long before chemotherapy was introduced. It is now known that purple grapes have at least 12 molecules that can safely kill cancer cells.

I wondered if it was the actual process of writing that produces a finished book or project. Then I concluded that it was the writing that produces the healing. By putting my traumas into language, whether written or spoken, people could come to a clear understanding of what had happened. I thought it best to write in a manner that a youth could understand what I was saying, as I hoped it would stop confusion. Trying to add meaning to a work is important even if the meaning is translated differently by various people.

Everyone, has at some time or some form or another, been affected by the scourge of cancer. What choices did these people make? The obvious choice is to overcome the cancer while you are still alive! It is amazing how much humour can keep people alive, simply by engaging in its life-saving energy. This harbours the question: what is the meaning of life?

Purposefulness, intentionality, and single-mindedness all combine to make one want to jump out of bed in the morning. All of these ingredients unite to make one want to fall asleep at night. It's what one loves and can't live without. It can be a job, a goal, a person, or anything that one is passionate about. My purpose, my intentionality, is to help others by spreading a positive message, to always make a smile contagious, and to assist wherever I possibly can. Without intention, there is no identity, no meaning to live. We are all given a purpose. What is the meaning of life? It's an ambiguous question with seven billion opinions, but it can be answered in a few words: Life is what YOU make it!

It's never too early or too late to find one's purpose in life. The time is now to answer the following questions as honestly as possible.

1. If you couldn't possible fail, what would you do?
2. What do you want the words on your tombstone to say? Remembering, of course, this simplifies what you truly value.
3. What do you really want your obituary to state? Summarising your wanted accomplishments, you will realise what goals you are so passionate about.
4. If you had to spend twenty-fours doing one thing, what would that be? This will possibly reveal the hobby you are obsessed with.
5. What must you do before you pass away? (The bucket list will make you ponder on this long-term).

When one has been diagnosed with cancer it is a shock to the victim's whole system. It is all too easy to resign to one's fate and sit in a chair and feel sorry for oneself, just waiting to die! The question that arises in nearly everyone's mind is, "Why me?" Cancer doesn't care for any person, male or female, child or adult!

This is where the power of positive thought can override any negative feelings. The cognitive powers of each and every one of us can manifest healing if only the suggestion can be registered in the first place!

Of course, there are numerous stories that abound regarding people surviving cancer that attempt to offer hope to patients who are currently undergoing whatever treatments. There are also many alternative treatments that are extremely expensive, too! It is only natural for anyone who has finished a cancer treatment to be concerned about what their future may hold. Many survivors have fears about the way they look, feel and about whether the cancer will eventually return. Other people are deeply concerned about what they can do, or learn, in an attempt to stop their cancer from returning. Understanding what to expect after cancer treatment can help those survivors and their families plan for follow-up care, make lifestyle changes, stay hopeful, and make important decisions.

All cancer survivors should have some type of follow-up care. They may have a great number of questions with regard to the care they need now, such as:

- Whether to tell the aftercare nurses about symptoms that worry them
- Which doctors/oncologists to see after treatment
- How often to see the doctor/oncologist.
- What specific tests they may require.
- What they can do to relieve pain and other problems after treatment.
- How long it will take for patients to recover from orthodox treatment and feel more like themselves again, if ever.

Dealing with these issues, and others, can be quite a challenge. Yet, many cancer patients say that becoming involved in decisions about their future medical care and lifestyle is a good way to regain some of the control they felt they lost during their cancer treatment. Research has shown that cancer patients, who feel more in control, feel and function better than those who do not. Being an active partner with your doctor and Palliative Care people may be the first step.

Remember, your body has been through a great ordeal. Therefore, allow your brain the opportunity to improve the immune system and heal the body. But, don't go rushing back into what was your previous lifestyle! Even a year from now will be too soon for some patients. No patient wants to overdo things and relapse and become bedridden again. Consider how best you can help heal your body, and the best way to do that is to relax and then relax even further and breathe plenty of FRESH air whenever you can, for at least half an hour every day! Cancer does not like fresh air!

(1). Cancer statistics, 2008, CA Cancer, J. Clin. 2008, 58, 71-96.

1
Living With Hope

Life is unfair! That maybe so, but all too often life is also a paradox because of a lack of hope. How many times did the outcomes we had planned or hoped to accomplish in life never became a reality. Our dreams, which are made with threads of hope, simply unravel and we are left pondering: "Is there really any hope, after all?"

All around us, people are in need of hope—genuine hope; the homeless, hospice patients, the unemployed, those who are desperately lonely, and cancer sufferers—people from all walks of life that are faced with circumstances, some medical, and thus, beyond their control. These people have little to cling to, except hope. Hope is the belief that in the future personal situations will get better. Without hope, there is the strong possibility that people sink into depression and despair.

Psychological development in, and interaction with a social environment, are supportive hope programs, especially in Canada, that have been found to increase quality of life and improve the personal health of persons with advanced cancer[1]. Since hope has been identified as a key psychological development resource among family caregivers to manage and deal with the caregiver experience[2-4], it is theorised that they may also benefit from a hope-focused intervention that is measured to their needs. Hope is, therefore, defined by family caregivers, as the inner strength to achieve future good and to continue caregiving[2].

Nevertheless, there are two aspects to the human side of cancer: what cancer does psychologically to people and their families, and how emotions, behaviours and incorrect nutrition may influence the risk of the development of cancer and its generally negative outcome.

Many cancer sufferers ask their medical practitioner: "Can you advise me which books, or articles, to read in order to help me cope better and get through this?"

I should think that query would be difficult to respond to because there are many books on coping with cancer. But many of those types of books tout a particular approach and promise that it alone will lead to successful coping.

If I have learned anything in this life, it is that there is no single correct approach and no simple solution that all cancer sufferers will agree with, especially when it comes to accepting proven findings in dealing with the human side of cancer. Although there are given universal testimonies about the cancer experience, particularly in the sense of uncertainty that people feel, we are each as distinct from one another in our psychological dimension as we are in the pattern of our fingerprints and our DNA. It is difficult to comprehend, given this diversity, that there is only one correct answer for every cancer sufferer.

However, when a cancer sufferer's alternative treatment is categorised as a miracle by orthodox medicine, then perhaps, we all need to reappraise our present thinking on cancer treatment! There is more than one correct solution and one series of treatments, other than surgery, radiation therapy and chemotherapy.

· · · ·

You may have just been informed that you have a particular type of cancer, or you may already be undergoing treatment and feel a complete loss of hope. Perhaps, you are a cancer survivor, wondering whether you are cured, or not. Or you are coping with cancer as a chronic disease and feel the need for mental support. Maybe, you are a home caregiver on the cancer journey, supporting and assisting a loved one with cancer, but feeling the need for help yourself.

Whatever your situation, I would like to be able to sit with you and talk about what's been going on and how you've been coping, and attempt to help you find the kind of support that suits just you! That's the way I would like to do it. But since that's impossible, I've tried through the chapters of this book to talk with people as if we were talking face-to-face about their illness or that of their loved one and about the problems they have had to deal with travelling the cancer journey.

I have heard many a "cancer journey," starting with find-ing a lump or having a pain that resulted in a visit to the doctor, who, finally, diagnosed cancer. Or, for others, it is how they were suddenly and completely surprised by the results of a routine mammogram or colonoscopy or chest X-ray that showed early signs of cancer. Somewhere along the journey, each has heard a version of the words: "I am sorry, but you have been diagnosed with cancer."

Some people, when they hear this news become scared, mixed up, and overwhelmed to the point that they hesitate to take the next step. Others come later, such as after starting their chosen type of cancer treatment. Then they hit the "Loss of Hope" syndrome as they attempt to cope with surgery, radiation and chemotherapy. The loss of hope syndrome starts with feelings that lead to questions such as: Can I get through this? Is there a light at the end of the tunnel? Have I undergone all of this orthodox treatment, feeling constantly nauseous and losing all of my hair . . . for nothing?

Whatever their situation, cancer sufferers need to talk about how difficult it has been to get to where they are now. They often have only looked at their personal shortcomings in meeting the day-to-day crises, seeing only the trees and not the forest. They need to focus more on the bigger picture, which so many times reveal just how remarkably strong and courageous they have been in the face of one of life's gravest challenges: the threat to life itself.

Sometimes, it is not the person with cancer who seeks advice, but rather a family member or other loved one who finds it painful to watch as the person encounters the highways and byways of the cancer journey.

Cancer sufferers need to look at their inner sources of strength, and identify their well-honed ways of dealing with adversity that has worked in the past and, with restoration in the power of hope, will work again. They also need to discover what they know, and don't know, about their particular cancer and what they really need to know about the alternative cancer treatments that are out there in the world and which, have been proven to be successful!

Each and every person suffering from cancer brings unique characteristics to dealing with their own illness: a particular personality, a way of coping, a set of beliefs and values, a way of looking at the world; a genuine desire to trust in hope! The goal is to take these qualities into consideration and make sure that they work in their favour at each point along the cancer journey.

I implore cancer sufferers to make their own cancer journey easier and keep from losing all hope. For without some degree of hope, there is absolutely nothing!

Some cancer sufferers can offer their experience to the medical profession, sharing their experiences and exploring the personal meaning that cancer had in their lives. The medical profession can learn how to identify those who are distressed, who need support and help. Then and only then, can the medical profession begin to understand what the common problems are and how to help the cancer sufferer deal with them.

Living without any kind of genuine hope is no life at all!

References:
(1). Duggleby W, Degner L, Williams A, Wright K, Cooper D, Popkin D, et al.: *Living with Hope: Initial evaluation of a psychosocial hope intervention for older palliative home care patients.* *Journal of Pain and Symptom Management* 2007, 33(3):247-57. PubMed Abstract | Publisher Full Text.

(2). Holtslander L, Duggleby W, Williams A, Wright K: *The experience of hope for informal caregivers of palliative patients.* *Journal of Palliative Care* 2005, 21(4):285-91. PubMed Abstract.

(3). Herth K: *Hope in the family caregiver of terminally ill people.* *Journal of Advanced Nursing* 1993, 18:538-48. PubMed Abstract Publisher Full Text.

(4). Borneman T, Stahl C, Ferrell B, Smith D: *The concept of hope in family caregivers of patients at home.* *Journal of Hospice and Palliative Nursing* 2002, 4(1):21-33. Publisher Full Text.

2

Accepting the Inevitable

My local MD informed me that the biopsy taken of the lump in my shoulder/neck area was, indeed, a melanoma and needed to be surgically removed as soon as possible. He handed me a referral note for the melanoma cancer surgery specialist at the Mater Private Clinic. I attended the specialist skin cancer surgeon's office three weeks later. Dr. Chris Allen was friendly and assured both Jeannie and I that he had successfully performed numerous such operations. After studying his notes, he looked up, smiled, and said: "This is the first time I've had a patient who's been mauled by a man-eating tiger! That must have been some experience!"

"I have been told it was a unique event," I replied.

Dr. Allen then went on to explain about melanoma. He emphasised that it was most difficult, if not impossible, to ascertain where the melanoma cells go when the cancer metastacises, or spreads. PET scans cannot detect the exact whereabouts of these minute cancer cells. Even after a period of no signs of melanoma cancer it can reappear at any time, and anywhere. That is why melanoma is considered to be the most dangerous of all cancers.

Dr. Allen further told us that he would have a colleague assisting with this four and a half hour surgery operation; a surgeon most experienced in this field. I began to feel more comfortable as Dr. Allen's manner and friendly attitude certainly helped ease our tensions.

After the operation I was surprised to find that besides a small scar on my neck, I also had a much larger scar on the right-hand side of my neck. On attending Dr. Allen's next appointment after the operation, Jeannie and I were told the surgery had been a success and, as a matter of procedure, twenty lymph nodes had been removed to ascertain if any cancer cells were evident in that area. The doctor smiled as he said that the removed lymph nodes were free of any cancer. I breathed a sigh of relief.

During the four-and-a half hour operation my arm was placed in an awkward position, causing my rotator cuff to be damaged, leaving it with two tears. It was painful and physiotherapy was advised, but only an initial treatment was activated as more melanomas appeared in the area. Surgery on the melanoma tumour was considered more important than physiotherapy treatment for the damaged rotator cuff.

Some weeks later I noticed another lump in the same area. I phoned Dr. Allen for an appointment and was allocated one almost immediately. A biopsy was taken and it was found that this lump, too, was a melanoma. Dr. Allen showed complete surprise by the result and admitted that he was disappointed by the findings. A new surgery appointment was made for the following week. This operation, too, was successful.

Three weeks later, and to my utter disappointment, I found yet another lump in the same area! I pondered deeply about the significance of the lymph nodes being declared clear, when there wasn't supposed to be any cancer cells present! Jeannie phoned for an appointment, which was made for the end of that week.

On entering his office, Dr. Allen looked very concerned as he intimated that if these lumps continued to appear he would need to consult with colleagues with the possibility of having radiation therapy in this area. I was none too happy with this suggestion but I accepted the inevitable, as the chemotherapy procedure was regarded as inefficient for melanoma cancer.

Needless to say, yet a further lump appeared within another three week period. I was processed for radiation therapy, which consisted of twenty treatments to be performed every day, except on the weekends. I was informed that because the radiation unit had over 170 patients per day it was impossible to have appointments to always suit the patient. This was unfortunate for me, as I lived on Macleay Island in the Morton Bay area. Therefore, my appointments for radiation ranged from 8 a.m., through to 4 p.m.

All of the staff at the radiation department were polite and caring. I was made aware of the process of processing a thermoplastic face mask for my protection from radiation. It was an exact procedure, with a pliable sheet of plastic placed over my face and pressed into place. A week or so later I returned to this department to be fitted with my mask. I found the now rigid face mask tight-fitting and for some patients this could be claustrophobic. However, I felt no discomfort at all. The front of the face mask was tightly screwed into place on to a backboard. This was a different situation as to discomfort and this procedure really made the mask fit tight and it took several moments to come to terms with the close-fitting sensation. This face mask was worn each and every time I undertook radiation therapy.

During one therapy course something went amiss as I was left on the procedure table far longer than on previous occasions. The look of embarrassment on the attendant's face told me its own story . . . that something was not quite right, although nothing was offered as an explanation to me for the lengthy time lapse. Later, I suffered extreme pain in my neck area and it was explained that the myelin sheathing protecting the nerves in my neck had been melted by radiation, leaving the nerves permanently exposed with continuous extreme pain. Even though pharmaceutical medication was offered to help relieve the pain it was insufficient to ease my pain level. It was later explained that there was no remedy.

Finally, the radiation therapy treatment was completed. Then it was decided I have a CT scan of my whole body to ascertain what was happening on the inside. Just prior to my having the CT scan, I found yet another lump, still in the same area. I phoned Dr. Allen with my news. He suggested we wait for the CT scan results before further surgery.

The CT scans showed the worst possible result. The cancer had metastacised to other parts of my body, namely both lungs and the liver, with a mass of tumours in my neck. I began to wonder why the surgeon was even bothering to remove the latest tumour on my neck, when he knew my prognosis stated I had up to six months to live!

While stitching up the wound, Dr. Allen explained that "there were so many melanoma tumours in the area that it was impossible to remove them all! He strongly cautioned me that if any further lumps appeared, I was to get in contact with him immediately and he would arrange to remove them. He warned that if the tumours broke through the skin of their own accord, "they would make a horrible mess, which should be avoided at all costs."

My MD telephoned for Jeannie and I to make an urgent appointment. He went on to inform Jeannie and I that I had reached stage IV melanoma cancer!

I had always tried to look at the positive aspects of life at all costs, but on hearing this statement and realising I had been given a death sentence, I reached the lowest ebb in all of my life, which included being mauled by the tiger!

I asked how long I had to live and was informed "up to six months!"

I pondered on the value of being grateful for small mercies. I reflected on that point, as being the single most effective way to change my vibrations from negative to positive. In fact, gratitude and love are the very highest vibrations in the universe, and when you emit them, you will undoubtedly get them back ten-fold. Therefore, when standing in a long line waiting for service, or rushing home from work to prepare dinner for guests, try to remember to be grateful for whatever you can find to be grateful for in that moment, because the smallest things that you can think of, will shift your energy from negative to positive and that positive thought will attract more, and more, and more.

Therefore, what are some of the small things in your life that you appreciate and love? My list runs something like this: my grandchildren's future, family activities, muffins in the oven, dark chocolate, laughter, good music, eyes that smile, a refreshing beverage with a friend, a funny e-mail, a good book, sunshine on my face and, hoping the car will start first time!

I can think of many more instances and I know that you can, too! Just focus on one or two of your favourites as you stand there feeling harried, hassled and harassed and make sure to include random acts of kindness sent your way or sent by you! Random acts of kindness can start the wheel of gratitude spinning throughout your psyche, and as you help another, and send good vibes their way—giving them your best—for it truly is your best—you will find out that in giving, you are actually receiving.

You receive that warm fuzzy compassionate feeling that connects you to your source, your essence—your spirit within, that is the real you. And that is exactly what you need to do. You want to stay connected to your spirit, for it is the source of wisdom, peace and love. And when you can tap into that source with intentionality, you will be happier than you have been for a long while. By intentionally and genuinely giving to others, or by expressing thankfulness and appreciation in any way, shape or form, you will be receiving what you are giving out. It is a circle. It blesses both the giver and the receiver. And guess what else it is? It is evidence of the circular nature, or put more colloquially, evidence that "whatever comes around goes around."

Medical literature is full of facts about the effects of stress on our bodies. Lesser known studies now show that grateful people demonstrate higher levels of energy, enthusiasm, attentiveness and determination.

Therefore, deliberately choosing to feel grateful is a good thing! In fact, it is a sane and most wonderful way to live your life, on purpose, and with purpose, because the only real purpose of human life is to experience happiness. And choosing a few minutes a day while waiting at a traffic light or walking to your car to quieten your mind and feel grateful helps you develop a happy habit—a habit of controlling your thoughts and gaining mastery over negativity.

When I was at my lowest point, I remembered something very important! The fact that I was still alive and I could fight back against this horrible disease was a thought that registered in my mind. It was like a breath of fresh air! There had to be a way to fight back. I might not know of the answer immediately, but, sooner rather than later, an answer would arrive, all because of my positive attitude.

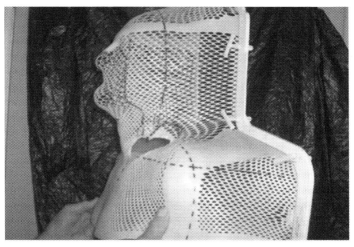

Side View of My Thermoplastic Face Mask.
The large hole was the area where the radiation entered.
(Photo: Author's Private Collection)

I knew that my sources of finding someone who was willing to even talk on this subject of cancer was more than a challenge, as people, for one reason or another can't seem to talk to cancer sufferers. They appear distant and embarrassed. Just a word of hello would have been nice! Personal friends certainly have their limitations. On the other hand, it was a pleasant experience meeting hospital volunteers who approached me with an open and caring attitude, willing to chat with me on any and every subject desired. It was such a comfort to me. You know who you are . . . thank you, so much!

::

"If the smallest part of the spirit suffers,
it imparts suffering to the whole body."
All too often many doctors have
seen this principle at work.

3
Understanding Melanoma Cancer

Let there be no misunderstanding that the sudden, mind-numbing announcement by the medical fraternity that you have cancer is not necessarily a death sentence! Practitioners are only offering their opinion based on orthodox practises, which include surgery, radiation therapy and chemotherapy, claiming that these are the only proven methods of eradicating cancer. The mere mention of the word cancer is enough to start one's heart racing, simply because of the word cancer.

I didn't survive the announcement of that death sentence completely unscathed. The prognosis that I had up to six months to live was certainly akin to being trapped in a deep dark cave, with no way of escape. I have never seen stalactites, or stalagmites, and I still cannot remember which ones hang down, and which ones stand up. Yet, in that dark place everything seemed to be topsy-turvy. I felt as if I was deep down without much hope of an alternative . . . deep down with me, my smidgeon of hope kept reminding me that what I had been told was a false statement, a misinterpretation, even a lie; call it what you will, but I simply knew the statement of the death sentence wasn't true. Accepting that hope can set you free from the fear of having cancer is only the beginning. People need to believe that that fear is not real. It never has been and never will be! It only exists in the mind of those who are not aware of the true, full facts. These types of people may seem to be alive but they are usually mentally dead, because they believe in the lie that cancer mostly wins out, killing its victims! However, from hope springs life anew!

How often has the phrase, "Take time to smell the flowers!" been bandied about? You don't have to smell the flowers, but perceive the stillness of those same flowers. Notice the stillness that derives from Peace, Perfect Peace! Listen to the silence all around you whenever you can. Notice it! Pay attention to it, for you will soon release yourself from the helter-skelter, rambunctious world and you will soon become aware of that dimension of inner silence within you.

Hope! Simply by trusting in hope brings with it an awareness that you are NOT who you think you are. You are not the real you! In that moment of noticing silence all around you, you are completely aware, yet, not thinking, entering into the dimension of inner silence of Perfect Peace, where the real you came from. This silence calms the mind, especially when confronted with an announcement that you have cancer and all the ramifications that that arouses!

It was hope that set me searching for my solution. I guess that the will to survive is stronger than people really imagine. Desperation can add to the willingness to survive, giving strength not to fall into the hands of panic, but rather to panic more slowly. I personally knew of no one who had survived from the scourge of cancer, yet that didn't hamper my eagerness to find something, someone, to give me some guidance.

My mind were not prepared for the startling announcement that I only had six months to live, which left me discombobulated; all the same, I was still conscious of a host of emotions, which flooded me: disorientation, shock, disbelief, anger, guilt, depression and fear, being a few examples. But uppermost was the strong notion not to panic, thereby losing control.

Experiencing these kinds of feelings is not felt just by the individual, for it is all too common in society. Learning to live with any type of cancer is not at all easy. There are no easy paint-by-numbers answers with this challenge. People may very well feel frightened and isolated. However, it is important to try and balance those delicate feelings so that you do not become utterly overwhelmed with numerous continuous negative thoughts.

One proactive method you can achieve with these feelings is to talk honestly with someone you trust implicitly. Sharing worries and fears is an important step in understanding and putting them in perspective. From my point of view, talking honestly certainly helps! The mere act of sharing and communicating can be a great release, however, it may be that you find it difficult to talk openly with those close to you about how you are coping with this new reality. You may feel that no one completely understands your particular anxieties and fears for the future. Or you may feel unable to talk freely about aspects of your care and future with your close family, even your spouse, and friends. If so, it may be useful to talk to someone who is either professionally experienced or who has experienced the very same challenge as yourself.

There are also a number of organisations which offer help such as:

- Pastoral care
- A priest
- Minister or member of a religious organisation
- District nurses
- Social workers
- Counselling organisations and support groups

One helpful strategy that I took on board was to obtain as much information as I could about my own particular type of cancer; what I was to expect and what I could do to help myself through it. Understanding my cancer and what my alternative treatment entailed went a long way to removing the mystery about the disease that enabled me to feel more in control. Attitude was extremely important; combined with positive and powerful thinking; as well as planning a well-balanced diet, learning relaxation techniques and taking regular exercise and breathing deeply that enabled me to actively participate in my treatment and recovery. Complementary therapies such as reflexology, aromatherapy and massage can help cancer sufferers to relax and, in doing so, improve their morale and ability to cope with the journey ahead.

I initially intended to keep a cancer dairy, but I became overwhelmed with all that was happening, therefore, I delayed keeping a record of my details, much to my annoyance later on. Cancer and its subsequent treatment may well inhibit your sexuality; in other words, how you feel about yourself as a man or a woman. Cancer treatments, especially orthodox practices, can cause vomiting, tiredness, irritability, pain, bowel problems and a general loss of energy. In addition, the repercussions of the emotional stresses of having cancer treatment should not be underestimated. Changes in body image as a result of scars, weight loss/gain, or the absence of a breast, for example, will also have an impact and all together may mean that for a time your interest in sex diminishes. Under such stressful circumstances, being able to talk openly with your partner will be very helpful in acknowledging worries and fears for the future. There are many alternative ways to feel loved, such as touch and massage—even a kind, comforting word. These can help reduce anxiety and depression and enable the cancer sufferer to feel more positive.

The experience of a cancer diagnosis and treatment will inevitably have a huge impact on many aspects of your life. It certainly did with me! However, I gave my cognitive abilities sufficient time to adjust and remembered that there were strategies that could help my life in the future. Be reassured that you are not alone and there is help, if you need it.

On a personal level, to find some kind of satisfactory answer to what melanoma cancer really meant, I turned to the Internet and I have used that source as an explanation. Wikipedia, a free encyclopaedia, provided information to help me and everyone else understand what was going on.

"All cancers are caused by damage to the DNA inside cells. This damage can be inherited in the form of genetic mutations, but in most cases, it builds up over a person's lifetime and is caused by factors within their environment. DNA damage causes the cell to grow out of control, leading to a tumour. Melanoma is usually caused by damage from UV light from the sun, yet, UV light from sunbeds is also said to be a contributing factor to the disease[1].

"The earliest stage of melanoma starts when the melanocytes begin to grow out of control. Melanocytes are found between the outer layer of the skin (the epidermis) and the next layer (the dermis). This early stage of the disease is called the radial growth phase, and the tumour is less than 1 mm thick. Because the cancer cells have not yet reached the blood vessels lower down in the skin, it is very unlikely that this early stage cancer will spread to other parts of the body. If the melanoma is detected at this stage, then it can usually be completely removed by surgery.

"When the tumour cells start to move in a different direction—vertically up into the epidermis and into the papillary dermis—the behaviour of the cells changes dramatically[2].

"The next step in the evolution is the invasive radial growth phase, which is a confusing term; however, it explains the next step in the process of the radial growth, when individual cells start to acquire invasive potential. This step is important—from this point on the melanoma is capable of spreading. The long-term outcome from malignant melanoma depends on its thickness, which is called the Breslow thickness. The Breslow's depth of the lesion is usually less than 1 mm (0.04 in), the Clark Level is usually two. To explain Breslow thickness and Clarke's Levels, both are measurements of the vertical height of the tumour in the skin. Tumour thickness is directly related to prognosis because thicker tumours have greater access to lymph capillaries, which is the usual method of spreading.

"Breslow thickness is measured in millimetres, whereas, the Clarke's Level describes depth relative to other skin structures and is now a less commonly used measure.

"The following step in the process is the invasive melanoma—the vertical growth phase (VGP). The tumour attains invasive potential, meaning it can grow into the surrounding tissue and can spread around the body through blood or lymph vessels. The tumour thickness is usually more than 1 mm (0.04 in), and the tumour involves the deeper parts of the dermis.

"The host elicits an immunological reaction against the tumour (during the VGP)[3], which is judged by the presence and activity of the tumour infiltrating lymphocytes (TILs). These cells sometimes completely destroy the primary tumour; this is called regression, which is the latest stage of the melanoma development. In certain cases, the primary tumour is completely destroyed and only the metastatic tumour discovered. Metastatic means spreading.

"A number of rare mutations, which often run in families, are known to greatly increase one's susceptibility to melanoma. Several different genes have been identified as increasing the risk of developing melanoma. Some rare genes have a relatively high risk of causing this disease; some more common genes, such as a gene called MC1R that causes red hair, have a relatively low risk. Genetic testing can be used to determine whether a person has one of the currently known mutations.

"Two-gene models of melanoma risk have already been created[4], and in the future, researchers hope to create genome-scale models that will allow them to predict a patient's risk of developing melanoma based on his or her genotype.

"In addition to identifying high-risk patients, researchers want to identify high-risk lesions (abnormal area of tissue) within a given patient. Many new technologies, such as Optical Coherence Tomography (OCT), are being developed to accomplish this. OCT allows pathologists to view three-dimensional reconstructions of the skin and offers more resolution than past techniques could provide. In vivo confocal microscopy and fluorescent tagged antibodies are also proving to be valuable diagnostic tools.

"In July 2009, the International Agency for Research on Cancer released a report that categorised tanning beds as "carcinogenic to humans". The agency, which is part of the World Health Organisation (WHO), previously classified tanning beds as "probably carcinogenic". The change comes after an analysis of more than 20 epidemiological studies indicating that people who begin using tanning devices before age 30 are 75% more likely to develop melanoma[5].

"Melanoma is a malignant tumour of melanocytes. Melanocytes are cells that produce the dark pigment, melanin, which is responsible for the colour of the skin. They predominantly occur in skin, but are also found in other parts of the body including the bowel and the eye (uveal melanoma is cancer of the eye.) Melanoma can occur in any part of the body that contains melanocytes.

"This horrible disease is less common than other skin cancers. However, it is much more dangerous and causes the majority (75%) of deaths related to skin cancer[6]. Worldwide, doctors diagnose about 160,000 new cases of melanoma yearly. The diagnosis is more frequent in women than in men and is particularly common among Caucasians living in sunny climates, with higher rates of incidence in Australia, New Zealand, North America, Latin America, and Northern Europe[7].

According to a World Health Organisation report, about 48,000 melanoma related deaths occur worldwide per year[8].

"The treatment includes surgical removal of the tumour, adjuvant treatment, (an additive that enhances the effectiveness of medical treatment), chemo—and immune-therapy, or radiation therapy. The chance of a cure is greatest when the tumour is discovered while it is still small and thin, and can be entirely removed surgically."

As for myself, I had seven surgical operations to remove the melanoma tumours in my neck. With each new surgery

I became more positive that surgery wasn't the complete answer. Yet, at that stage I was offered no other treatment. I was informed by a specialist that chemotherapy was of no use in my situation as chemotherapy is perhaps, successful in only three per cent of melanoma tumours.

1. Solar and Ultraviolet Radiation. IARC monographs on evaluation of carcinogenic risks to humans. 55, 1992.
2. Hershkovitz L, Schachte J, Treves AJ, Besser MJ (2010) "Focus on adoptive T cell transfer trials in melanoma." Clin. Dev. Immunal 2010: 260267. doi, 10. 1155/2010/260267. PMC. 3018069. PMID 21234353.
3. American Society of Clinical Oncology Annual Meeting Proceedings, Part 1, Abstract: Protective effect of a brisk tumour infiltrating lymphocyte infiltrate in melanoma: "A European Organisation for Research and Treatment of Cancer Melanoma Group Study." Journal of Clinical Oncology 25(185): 8519. 2007.
4. News Medical. "Melanoma Symptoms and Cause." Creative Commons Attribution—A Like Licence. Wikipedia.
5. WHO International Agency for Research on Cancer, Monograph Working Group, Aug 2009. "A Review of Human Carcinogens, Part D: Radiation." The Lancet Oncology 10(8), 751-2, doi: 10.16/s1470-2045(09) 70213.
6. Jerant AF, Johnson JT, Sheridan CD, Caffrey TJ (July 2000). "Early Detection and Treatment of Skin Cancer." Am Fam Physician. 62(2): 367-68, 375-6, 381-2. BMID 10929700.
7. Parkin D, Bray F, Ferlay J, Pisani P (2005). "Global Cancer Statistics, 2002." CA Cancer J Clin. 55(2): 75-8.
8. Lucas, R, McMichael T, Smith W, Armstrong B (2006) (pdf). "Solar Ultraviolet Radiation." Environmental Burden of Disease Series (3) WHO. ISBN 92 4 1594403.

4

Stage IV
Melanoma Cancer

When one hear the words "stage IV cancer," many things run through one's mind. "This is very likely to kill me," is just one of them!

Needless to say, my mind was in overdrive racing from one thought to another. Panic was now knocking at my brain. Panic slowly, I told myself. You can survive this! You've survived the tiger attack and being swept out to sea . . . so, you can and will survive this! I took a deep breath and the realisation came that there must be others who have been/are in the same situation as myself . . . I needed to find them! Or just one cancer survivor! Suddenly, a word came to mind—Internet! Yes! Of course! I discussed this brainstorm of an idea with Jeanne. She smiled and said nothing for a moment or two. Then she said:

"I do actually know of someone who may be able to help us! There's this man on Facebook . . . Vernon, an American. He's a genuine cancer survivor, who used an alternative treatment, and he has a website . . . I'll look it up!"

A few minutes later, Jeanne handed me a written website: www.pHkillscancer.com. This site now takes you to: "Vernon's Dance With Cancer". I rushed to my CP and typed in the website. I found the contact details easily enough and e-mailed Vernon with my desperate plea for more information about his personal recipe for the treatment of cancer. I wasn't certain that I would even get a reply, but Vernon replied almost immediately with the details.

To say I was astonished when I read one of the ingredients was bicarbonate of soda (baking soda), is the understatement of the year! Bicarbonate of soda, I knew, was a household word for a general cleansing agent around the house, including teeth! I had to think seriously about this alternative cancer treatment some more! Was Vernon playing a weird joke?

I waited a few hours, pondering about this treatment, somewhat wary. Then I came to the conclusion that people, told by the medical fraternity that there is no hope of recovery, and have taken the alternative treatment journey, then, surely, they would be the last people to play a joke on anyone! No! These survivors . . . these casualties of the Cancer War would never lie to anyone who is in the same situation as themselves!

With that thought still fresh in my mind, I bought a packet of Bicarbonate of Soda from the local food market. I also added a jar of blackstrap molasses, which was also part of the recipe. As I left the shop, I felt grateful that Vernon had passed on his alternative treatment recipe! But, then, I thought . . . why not? I'd be willing to share this fabulous weapon with a fellow cancer sufferer!

I told my family right from the very beginning, "This is my choice, but I'm also taking this alternative treatment just as much as for you as for me! This treatment and Jeannie and I are going to beat this! I need your prayers, and I hope I have your trust in my judgment in this!"

Luckily, we are a family with a great sense of humour and we found plenty of humorous moments to help get us through the cancer journey. This is not the whole story. Through Facebook, I noticed a name . . . Curtis John Mitchell, who was born in September, two days before me, but, obviously many years later. I was at first taken aback, not so much as to his birthdate, but his name! I have two twin grandsons, named Curtis and Mitchell!

I had to contact this man and tell him of this coincidence. I very briefly mentioned my experience with the tiger, more for interest sake than anything else.

After about a week later I received a reply from Curtis John Mitchell. In the meantime, I had been taking the alternative treatment recipe for cancer, twice daily. Then Curtis' reply arrived:

"My father called me his little tiger. My life is a story and I live the book with most people telling me I should write it down, for it's quite a remarkable journey. I agree that there is no such thing as coincidence. Most of the vertebrae in my neck were removed so that my dura* could be sliced open and my spinal cord observed by a bunch of neurosurgeons, as there appeared to be a giant tumour growing and it was distending my spinal cord from t7 all the way up into my brain causing paralysis."

Via Con Dios, Mate!

Curtis . . . A Spiritual Warrior.

::

Periods of doubt started creeping forward. I was sure it was cancer's way of trying to distract me, but I realised how important being positive about the effect of the treatment could be. Therefore, if doubt started to rear its head at any stage I was prepared to remain positive and continue with the fight against cancer.

I think it best that I offer a brief explanation as to understanding pH and what it actually stands for. There is a greater expansion about this in chapter 15.

A high acidity level can become a dangerous condition that weakens all body systems, which is very common today. It gives rise to an internal environment conducive to disease, as opposed to a pH balanced environment, which allows normal body function necessary for the body to resist disease. A healthy body maintains adequate alkaline reserves to meet emergency demands. When excess acids must be neutralised, our alkaline reserves are depleted leaving the body in a weakened condition.

A pH balanced diet, according to many experts, is a vital key to health maintenance.

pH (potential of hydrogen) is a measure of the acidity or alkalinity of a solution. It is measured on a scale of 0 to 14—the lower the pH the more acidic the solution, the higher the pH the more alkaline (or base) the solution. When a solution is neither acid nor alkaline it has a pH of 7 which is neutral.

Water is the most abundant compound in the human body, comprising 70% of the body. The body has acid-alkaline (or acid-base) ratio called the pH which is a balance between positively charged ions (acid-forming) and negatively charged ions (alkaline-forming.) The body continually strives to balance pH. When this balance is compromised many problems can occur.

It is important to understand that I am not talking about stomach acid or the pH of the stomach. I am talking about the pH of the body's fluids and tissues which is an entirely different matter.

Testing your body's acidity or alkalinity is carried out by using diagnostic pH strips. It is recommended that you test your pH levels to determine if your body's pH needs immediate attention. By using pH test strips, you can determine your pH factor quickly and easily in the privacy of your own home. If one's urinary pH fluctuates between 6.0 to 6.5 in the morning and between 6.5 and 7.0 in the evening, your body is functioning within a healthy range. If your saliva stays between 6.5 and 7.5 all day, your body is functioning within a healthy range. The best time to test your pH is about one hour before a meal and two hours after a meal.

Here is what I initially used against my cancer: From your supplier, purchase a container of Diagnostic pH strips. There are approximately 90 strips in the package. Mine cost just short of $A21.00. Then, first thing in the morning, by the process of what is called a midstream sample, urinate on the strip. Shake of the residue off and wait a few seconds. This is the more reliable method, rather than using the saliva test as that process is not as consistent as the midstream urine method. Once you have found your pH level, say, 5.5, for example, this means your body is acidic and at a degree that cancer loves. The pH level for killing the cancer is pH 8.5.

To begin, take one level teaspoon of Bicarbonate of Soda (NOT Baking Powder!) and place it in a, say, medium-sized glass. Add one teaspoon of blackstrap molasses, mixing the two ingredients together with warm water. Drink this two hours before, or two hours after a meal—twice a day. Don't take more than three teaspoons of the bicarbonate of soda.

The next morning, when you have taken your urination sample, if the reading has not reached 8.5, then increase the Bicarbonate of Soda by one half, or another complete teaspoonful, making a total of two teaspoons for the bicarbonate of soda, but . . . do NOT increase the dosage of the molasses. Keep it always at one teaspoonful.

Continue adding the bicarbonate of soda until the pH reading is pH 8.5, then from that point on, return to one teaspoon of both the bicarbonate of soda and the molasses. But, don't forget the deep breathing strategy! I drank this recipe for ten consecutive days, just to be sure! Vernon drank it for five days as he had a CT scan appointment due. That scan, incidentally, showed he had no cancer in his body! However, the medical fraternity thought the scanning device was defective and made Vernon have another scan! The result was the same!

I also added extra items to the Treatment Plan in my fight against this melanoma cancer. Jeannie had purchased a "Champion" juicer, therefore, she immediately commenced juicing: carrots and beetroot together with pieces of ginger and one tablespoon of Barley Grass (in powder form) and a tablespoon of aloe vera juice, two apples and a stalk of celery, using the whole celery stalk and its leaves. This also was taken twice a day, usually at lunch time and at dinner time.

After the ten days of taking the Bicarbonate of Soda recipe, I thought . . . what next? Surely, this isn't all there is to it!

On a previous visit to the Eumundi Markets, Jeannie met the well-known Sunshine Coast naturopath and herbalist, Dominique Finney, BHsc., ND. Jeannie and Dominique soon struck up a firm friendship with Jeannie becoming a client almost immediately. When we realised that we needed the outside help of a naturopath, Jeannie immediately thought of Dominique. An e-mail was sent explaining my cancer situation, with a reply arriving the same day.

"Good to hear from you again, Jeannie. I know you have been busy painting and I congratulate you on your website, www.jeannefrost.com and your excellent abstract paintings! Say 'Hi' to Frank, also for me. As usual, I have been busy with my many clients and they certainly keep me busy. The satisfying aspect is that I have been receiving so many compliments on my various herbal treatments! Now, as to your email: I have worked with people in Frank's situation many times and am happy to help him with herbs, if he will take them! He needs to take 60 mls a day, which is two doses of 30 ml each or four doses of 15 ml each.

"Please, look these herbs up on the Internet and you will see why I pop them in the blender to strengthen his body. I am not able to make claims with cancer treatments. However, I do extract herbs that are associated with this and I am happy to mix them for him. The herbs are: *Carioca papaya* (paw paw extract); *Artemisia annua* (sweet annie) and *Juglan nigra* (black walnut hulls).

"I can put you in touch with previous clients if you need to read their testimonials about the effectiveness of supporting the body with these herbs. Frank will also need to have fresh juices daily. Also, as much as possible, delete out all wheat products completely from his diet.

"When taking the mixture, Frank may need to dilute the mixture slightly. After taking the mixture the next dosage should be in seven hours' time. I would suggest that Frank take his first dose at, say, ten a.m. And the next dose at five p.m. However, at lunch time, he should have a small portion of red meat (about enough to fill the palm of one hand) should suffice.

"With regards,

Dominique Finney."

I researched the ingredients on the Internet and this is what I found: *Carica papaya*. Paw paw is rich in enzymes called papain and chymopapain, which helps with the digestion particularly. It breaks down the proteins from food eaten into amino acids. The latest research shows that amino acids are responsible for all what is happening in our organism, basically for what is happening in every chemical reaction as well as our mental and physical health. As people age we produce less of the digestive enzymes in our stomach and pancreas, which leads to ineffective digestion of proteins. Due to this, people end up with excess amount of undigested protein, which leads to overgrowth of the bad bacteria in the gastro-intestinal system and not enough of amino acids to perform all important chemical reactions. It can be said that good quality protein is absolutely essential for people's healthy being. This is where the papaya enzymes can be very beneficial. The papain enzymes are produced in the skinny peel of paw paw. The combination of these enzymes repels insects during the ripening, without this protection paw paw fruit would not survive.

Eating paw paw after a meal certainly makes for better digestion; prevents bloating and chronic indigestion. It can also lower the inflammation in the body, alleviates the pain and oedema caused by sport injuries. Because of its anti-inflammatory properties papaya can relieve the severity of rheumatoid arthritis and osteoarthritis. Because of its high antioxidant content, papaya can prevent cholesterol oxidation and can be used in preventative treatments against athero-sclerosis, strokes, heart attacks and diabetic heart disease. In everyday health, papaya works magic on strengthening the immune system, preventing the recurrent colds and flu. After treatment with antibiotics, eating paw paw or drinking its juice replenishes the good intestinal bacteria, which was destroyed by the antibiotic treatment. The latest good news from eating paw paw, once again shows that papain, the enzyme which I talked about, was found to destroy intestinal parasites. Papain is a proteolitic enzyme, which means that it digests inert (non-living) proteins. Intestinal parasites are largely protein. The papain attacks it and causes any parasite to die. Also, home applications of leaf and bark papaya extract is used to deal with mouth gums and toothaches, which are being effectively practised in many cultures around the world.

Papain is also being studied for relief of cancer therapy side-effects, especially relieving side-effects such as difficulty in swallowing and mouth sores after radiation and chemo-therapy as well as boosting up the immune system and helping the body to fight the cancer.

I did, in fact, look up *artemisia annua* on the Internet. It is also known as Sweet Wormwood, Sweet Sagewort and Annua Wormwood. This is what I found: "The cancer-fighting potential of *artemisia annua* generated a great deal of interest in the herb, described in the ancient Chinese manuscript and used in many studies today."

I found this snippet: "*Antemisia annua* has also been shown to have anti-cancer properties. It is said to have the ability to be selectively toxic to some breast cancer cells [Cancer Research 65: Dec 1, 2005] and some form of prostate cancer. There have been exciting preclinical results against leukaemia, and other cancer cells."

Juglan nigra. Traditionally, black walnut has been used to fight cancer with some success, and this use has received some experimental support. The herb also has alterative, laxative, astringent, detergent, and hepatic properties. Its astringent uses, as a douche for leukor-rhea and a mouthwash for sores and inflammation, can be attributed to tannic acid. External applications can kill ringworm.

I made a determined decision to take whatever would help fight my cancer!

Into the bargain, I turned to one of the Japanese products called, miso. Now, there are several different types of this product, which results as a paste—after being fermented from anywhere up to two years! It can be made from rice or soya beans and makes a remarkable tasty drink or a soup. But why, *miso*?

I remembered something about the atomic bombing of Nagasaki and Hiroshima and *miso*. I had to check my memory on the Internet. This is what I found.

In his book, *Macrobiotic Diet*, Michio Kushi states: "At the time of the atomic bombing of Nagasaki in 1945, Tatsuichiro Akizuki, M.D., was director of the Department of Internal Medicine at St Francis Hospital in Nagasaki. Most patients in the hospital, located one mile from the centre of the blast, survived the initial effects of the bomb, but, soon after, came down with symptoms of radiation sickness from the radio-activity that had been released. Dr. Akizuki fed his staff and patients a strict macrobiotic diet of brown rice, *miso** and *tamari* soy sauce soup, *wakame* and other sea vegetables, Hokkaido pumpkin, and sea salt. Prohibited was the consumption of sugar and sweets. As a result, he saved everyone in his hospital, while many other survivors in the city perished from radiation sickness."

I was offered other forms of treatment, such as Reiki, meditation therapies, Violet Light, and long-distance healing, and energy healing. I accepted all treatments without the slightest negative thought . . . what did I have to lose, as according to the medical professionals, death was already knocking at my door? Of course, I was placed on prayer treatments, as well. I had to have the courage to accept whatever was offered in the way of treatment, help, call it what you will. I accepted willingly!

Each and every one of these treatments, I am sure, added to my healing. If any reader scoffs at this statement, I suggest they walk in my shoes for six months and find out from personal experience!

The alternative treatment journey is being made more aware by the public by the sheer truth that people are recovering from diagnoses of stage IV cancer. I must repeat, stage IV cancer is NOT necessarily a death sentence!

It's also important to find a cancer friend, someone who has been there, someone who knows and can understand your rawest emotions. This is where Vernon Johnston and Curtis John Mitchell fitted into my scenario. No cancer survivor will tell a cancer patient a lie! That is the whole truth of the matter!

Before my stage IV diagnosis, I led an average lifestyle. I was too busy all of the time! Now, I constantly live in the "now" moment-by-moment with a daily appreciation for every aspect of life. As Curtis John Mitchell said to me; "Enjoy the journey of cancer! The hardest part of the cancer journey is other people's beliefs. Be aware of them and how they limit you. That is when some people are able to move beyond the diagnosis of medical doctors when they believe they can. I found that breathing in fresh air deeply for at least half an hour a day was a great benefit. Cancer does not like fresh air!"

But, then again, cancer can be the worst thing that can ever happen to anyone. But, truthfully, from an inner perspective, it is also the best thing that has ever happened . . . to me or anyone else! It teaches you a great deal about yourself and about tolerance for one thing, and allows you to reflect on what is really important in one's life!

My cancer has had an impact on me in other ways. I began this book as an explanatory melanoma awareness story. I want to be involved in making everyone aware, giving hope to those who needed it, about melanoma and its affects. Unfortunately, many people think that melanoma is simply skin cancer, but, it can also kill you, or anyone else, before you even know you have it!

I am uncertain about the overall cancer war, but I'm working on it with the same attitude I adopted early on. I try not to allow cancer to interfere with my day, as I laugh at the absurdities of life. That's another thing about cancer, you soon realise what is important and what is not and you recognise that political correctness and political arguments are a load of complete nonsense. But, these days, things that used to irritate me, I merely laugh at, good and loud. Remember to deal with what is important, rather than what is considered urgent!

Cancer survivors all know this: You just don't know how strong you are until you walk away from a death sentence!

---

* Dura: The outermost, toughest, and most fibrous of the three membranes (meninges) covering the brain and the spinal cord.

* Miso: paste made from fermented soya beans and barley or rice malt, used in Japanese/macrobiotic cookery.

5
The Truth About Bicarbonate of Soda

There have been a great deal of misinformation published and gossiped about bicarbonate of soda and even doctors who advocate the usefulness of this product have been ridiculed; doctors such as Dr. Thomas P. Kennedy of the American Medical Association for one. Dr. Tullio Simoncini, an oncologist in Rome, Italy, has pioneered sodium bicarbonate (NaHCO3) therapy as a means to treat cancer, is another to face ridicule. Therefore, there is a need for some true facts about bicarbonate of soda to be revealed.

You may very well need to put your cognitive abilities into gear before you digest this article as your life may very well depend upon it! Although you have no rational reason to take my word for it, what about the word of a man who has been awarded a Nobel Prize—twice? If you were told the absolute truth about a substance and its use in the treatment of melanoma cancer, would you be able to grasp the significance of what you have been told? Possibly not! Especially when there is so much misinformation being bandied about by unscrupulous business concerns. Therefore, I would offer that it would be wise to take notice of the words of a respected doctor, who has spent much of his life studying cancer—and who has an open mind!

Doctors, such as Otto Warburg, twice a Nobel Prize recipient, and Mark Sircus, Ac, OMD, know a great deal about the fatal effects of bicarbonate of soda on cancer. Here then, are the true facts about bicarbonate of soda that the public would never have guessed. Even before finishing this article, people will be asking themselves why this valuable information has been suppressed for years! As a good example, I am living proof that the bicarbonate of soda and blackstrap molasses treatment are amalgamated with the miraculous findings with respect to metastacised melanoma cancer. My intentionality then is to offer this, and other information, to decide this issue once and for all.

The body's pH level is extremely important because pH controls the speed of the body's biochemical reaction. It does this by controlling the speed of the enzyme activity as well as the speed that electricity moves through our body.

The higher the pH level of a substance, or solution, the more electrical resistance that substance or solution holds. Therefore, electricity travels slower with higher pH. If something has an acidic pH, it is hot and fast. Alkaline pH on the other hand, biochemically speaking, is slow and cool. Cancer tissues have a much higher concentration of toxic chemicals, pesticides etc., than do healthy tissues. Part of any successful cancer treatment includes chelation and detoxification of heavy metals and a host of toxic chemicals, which are invading our body every day. Chelation (pronounced key-LAY-shun) is the use of a chemical substance to bind molecules such as metals or minerals and hold them tightly so they can be removed from the body. Chelation has been scientifically proven to remove excess or toxic metals before they can cause damage to the body.

Chelation was initially used in the 1940s by the United States Navy to treat lead poisoning. It is literally raining mercury; uranium contamination is increasing; lead, it has been discovered, is even more toxic than anyone ever believed and is in some bread products consumed by the public. Arsenic is in our chickens yet, most governments still want the public to receive their yearly mercury injection, dentists, of course, are still using hundreds of tons of mercury, exposing patients to internalised toxic waste dumps. Fluoride is still placed in the water supply and chlorine is breathed in from most people's home showers. This just covers a small slice of the toxic disaster that is the hallmark of life in the 21st century. It seems inconceivable to me that some oncologists have somehow, just not been able to comprehend that cancer patients are suffering from poisoning on a massive scale, with all the chemicals that scientists have already established, actually causing the cancer!

Hidden Knowledge

Otto Warburg, whose father was also a doctor, was born in 1883. Otto studied under a Nobel Prize winner who helped him advance in his understanding and knowledge in science regarding the cause of cancer, which led to his winning the Nobel Prize. He was awarded a second Nobel Prize, but he was unable to accept it during Adolf Hitler's Nazi regime, because he was of Jewish heritage. Basically, then, Otto Warburg won two Nobel Prizes for his discoveries about cancer.

When a doctor is nominated for a Nobel Prize for writing facts about cancer, then it can be honestly said that he certainly knows what he is talking about! Therefore, if a person wins two Nobel Prizes for cancer it should be doubly appreciated that he knows what he is talking about! Yet, science disagrees with such an eminent figure as Dr. Otto Warburg! Shouldn't someone investigate as to why this is?

About thirty years after being awarded his first Nobel Prize, Dr. Otto Warburg (a cell physiologist and biochemist) began working with Dr. Carl Reich on a part-time basis. However, Dr. Carl Reich never gave up and some twenty years later he and Robert Barefoot (biochemist) produced the book, *The Calcium Factor*. To simplify the research, Robert Barefoot wrote *Death by Diet* as he had enough knowledge to put the remaining pieces together.

It has to be realised that Dr. Warburg talks about enzyme deficiency with cooked foods. What basically happens with cooked food is that the enzymes are destroyed which, after ingestion, causes the red blood cells to cluster together.

Simply put, a normal red blood cell is seven microns in diameter. When a family is fed enzyme deficient foods the red blood cells are weakened and stick together in groups and can't travel through the smaller veins. This causes the body to have many low, or no oxygen areas, within the body, which allows cancer to develop. It is far better if your body is towards an alkaline level, then the cancer cannot continue to survive because your body is basically more oxygenated.

It is proven how important sulphur is in human health and how useful a basic chemical such as sodium thiosulphate* (Na_2SO_4) can be; now, people can get an instant course in the power of sodium bicarbonate and the act of instantly turning cancer cells alkaline. It is so effective that it is similar to shooting a guided cruise missile at them. That is how effective, safe, quick and precise bicarbonate of soda is, and it is inexpensive as well. Just a few days of bicarbonate of soda will keep cancer further away, keeping it at arm's length from ourselves, patients and loved ones. It is an ingredient that people can use to treat their water with as well, and excellent to put in distilled or reverse osmosis water or any water, for that matter.

Cancer basically needs a low oxygen environment to survive. Basically, 99% of the time, a terminal cancer victim's body is a thousand times more acidic than normal. Yet, both these environments are causing a low or non-oxygen environment which cancer loves. This is causing a low oxygen environment which means that many people are calcium deficient—and their cells are oxygen starved. This is why it is important to maintain a deep breathing exercise with fresh air every morning.

Dr. Warburg stated in his book, *The Metabolism of Tumours*, the primary cause of tumours was the replacement of oxygen in

---

*   Total consumption of Na_2SO_4 in Europe was around 1.6 million tons in 2001, of which 80% was used for detergents. However this use is waning, as domestic consumers switch to liquid detergents which do not include sodium sulphate.

the respiratory cell chemistry by the fermentation of sugar. The growth of cancer cells is initiated by a fermentation process, which can be trigged only in the absence of oxygen at the cell level. What Dr. Warburg was describing was a classic picture of acidic conditions. Just as when overworked muscle cells manufacture lactic acid by-products as waste, cancerous cells spill lactic acid and other acidic compounds causing acid pH.

Dr. Warburg states that a true conception of cancer was impossible without comprehending why some tissues in the body are deficient of oxygen and, therefore, prone to cancer. Cancerous tissues are acidic, whereas healthy tissues are alkaline. Water (H_2O) decomposes into H+ and OH-. When a solution contains more H+ and OH—then it is said to be acidic. When it contains more OH—than H+ ions then it is said to be alkaline. When oxygen enters an acid solution it can combine with H+ ions to form water. Oxygen helps to neutralise the acid, while at the same time the acid prevents oxygen from reaching the tissues that need it. Acidic tissues are devoid of free oxygen. An alkaline solution is just the reverse. Two hydroxyl ions (OH-) can combine to produce one water molecule and one oxygen atom. In other words, an alkaline solution can provide oxygen to the tissues.

The pH scale goes from 0 to 14, with 7 being neutral. Below 7 is acidic and above 7 is alkaline. The blood, lymph and cerebral spinal fluid in the human body are designed to be slightly alkaline at a pH of 7.4.

At a pH slightly above 7.4, cancer cells become dormant and at pH 8.5, cancer cells will die within hours, yet, healthy cells will live. This has given rise to a variety of treatments based on increasing the alkalinity of the tissues such as vegetarian diet, the drinking of fresh fruit juice and vegetable juices, and dietary supplementation with alkaline minerals, for instance: calcium, potassium, magnesium, cesium and rubidium. But, nothing can compare to the instant alkalising power of sodium bicarbonate for safe and effective treatment of cancer. Adding molasses to the recipe acts as an attractant to the cancer cells and then the bicarbonate of soda does its job killing off the cancer cells. However, deep breathing exercises of at least 20 minutes a day is a must!

Finally, a word or two about bicarbonate of soda. It comes from Dr. Thomas P Kennedy, of the American Medical Association.

"Sodium bicarbonate is a chemical compound with the formula $NaHCO_3$. Sodium bicarbonate (baking soda) is commonly used as an antacid for short-term relief of stomach upset, to correct acidosis in kidney disorders, to make the urine alkaline during bladder infections and to minimise uric acid crystallisation during gout treatment. Sodium bicarbonate is available as a non-prescription product as well as a general household item. It is also used with other non-prescription drugs for short term treatment of various conditions to treat anything from fever to moderate pain.

"Sodium bicarbonate possesses the property of absorbing heavy metals, dioxins and furans. Comparison of cancer tissue with healthy tissue from the same person shows that the cancer tissue has a much higher concentration of toxic chemicals, pesticides etc. Sodium bicarbonate neutralises acids present in gases (in particular, hydrochloric acid, sulphur dioxide, hydrofluoric acid) to form sodium salts (sodium chloride, sodium sulphate, sodium fluoride and sodium carbonate) which are all known as Residual Sodium Chemicals. Sodium bicarbonate can be made into a paste salve with vinegar. It relieves burning from bug stings (particularly bee stings), poison ivy, nettles, and sunburn. It is used as an antacid to treat acid in digestion and heartburn.

6

Differences of Opinion

Metastasis is a very high risk for anyone who has been treated for melanoma cancer. However, when the primary melanoma (original tumour) is thin (less than one millimetre in thickness), surgical removal offers a complete cure in 95% of patients, because the melanoma often, but not always, tends to be confined to the top layers of skin and is not likely to spread. This does not mean that one can be lax about self-examinations and check-ups. As 5% of thin melanomas are not always cured, it is extremely important to perform regular self-examinations of your skin and lymph nodes and keep all appointments for check-ups.

When your physician suspects that the melanoma may have spread, diagnostic testing will be conducted to determine if the cancer has spread and to where. Tests used to determine if the melanoma has spread include blood tests, X-rays, and imaging studies, including CT scans. Your dermatologist or oncologist should be able to determine which diagnostic tests are needed.

When melanoma cells spread from the primary tumour, they first pass through the lymph channel nearest to the melanoma. Once the melanoma has spread to the regional lymph nodes (the nodes nearest the tumour), there is a risk that the melanoma will spread to distant sites (other lymph nodes and organs). Once the melanoma has spread to distant sites, it has reached stage IV. Orthodox treatment of stage IV cancer may include selective surgical excision, radiation therapy, chemotherapy, and immune therapy. However, the prognosis is usually poor, and organ failure often causes death.

Moreover, it is important to know that more than "some" people do survive stage IV metastacised melanoma cancer. In stage IV cancer, melanoma can spread to organs in nearly every part of the body. Yet, cancer cells do not randomly shoot off in all directions. Each type of cancer (breast, pancreatic, prostate, etc.) has a strong likelihood of spreading to certain sites more often than others.

::

A Palliative Care team was allocated to Jeannie and I. A doctor and a nurse comprised our team which came to our home on the island to evaluate my condition and attitude and to measure Jeannie's stress level as well as her reactions to the situation.

The team were both polite and friendly, at first. The doctor's attitude changed after I asked his opinion about alternative treatments for cancer.

The doctor spoke firmly: "I shouldn't think it wise to contemplate any miracles happening. I am speaking from experience, you understand!"

"That may be, but I have heard a great deal about alternative treatments having numerous successes!" I countered.

"Nevertheless, orthodox medicine is the only proven method, which, in my opinion, is tantamount to curing cancer patients!" replied the doctor.

Jeannie gave the doctor a captivating smile and said: "Frank is overly concerned, as you will appreciate, Doctor, for he has been told that the medical profession can no longer do anything for him . . . would you like a cup of coffee, or tea, Doctor?"

I held my tongue from saying: "It is nigh impossible to get a medical practitioner to understand, as well as agree with something when his professional standing is dependent upon his not understanding or agreeing with it!"

However, in saying that, much later I met a newly-arrived doctor from Africa who was willing to listen and was keen to learn what I had taken to substantially improve my condition. Of course, this was after he had seen my two CT scans which had caused all the kerfuffle at the hospital.

However, the Palliative Care team were under no illusion about my diagnosis of stage IV melanoma cancer and that I had been given up to six months to live.

"You understand, Mr Burdett that we are here to make it understood that you will not suffer any tremendous discomfort as we will administer whatever medication is necessary to ease your comfort at all times," said the doctor.

Jeannie said nothing and neither did I.

The doctor continued: "It is our duty to care for cancer patients who have reached the stage where the medical profession can offer no help at this stage. There is no stage V, you understand. Please, feel free to ask any questions that may be troubling you and we will do our best to answer, within reason, of course!"

"I certainly understand my position, perfectly, Doctor. I have no questions at this stage but if I think of anything I will be in touch. Thank you for your comments. It must be disquieting for you to be in this position," I replied.

"Is there anything about your CT scans that you need explaining?" he asked.

"Not exactly, as being given up to six months to live is more than enough to digest at present!"

"The profession has had some wonderful successes with orthodox treatment, Mr Burdett, and new drugs are coming to the fore more than ever, so there is hope for some cancer sufferers, after all," he added.

"I do not wish to debate the pros and cons regarding cancer treatments, Doctor. I just want to concentrate on overcoming my present situation and continue with my alternative treatment, as the medical profession have given up on me!"

"As I have intimated before, Mr Burdett, it doesn't pay to rely too much on miracles!" he responded.

"We each have our opinions, Doctor. I can only try to fight this cancer the best way I think fit!"

"I wish you all the very best, Mr Burdett!" the doctor concluded.

7

"You Are Bleeding Internally!"

It was now ten months after I was supposed to have left the planet, during which, I had an appointment with my island MD. He looked at me and said: "You look rather anaemic. Are you feeling all right?"

"Yes! I feel a bit tired, but I feel all right!" I explained. "I have been digging in my raised garden beds for several hours a day and tidying up fallen palm leaves . . ."

"I think you are bleeding inside. I want you to have a blood test and I want you to start taking iron tablets!" said the MD.

I couldn't believe a word he had said. I felt tired, not run down and weak from loss of blood! I sat there saying nothing further. I duly had the blood test and I was asked to return and see the doctor within a couple of days.

"Yes, your iron level is down all right and I still think you are bleeding internally! I want you to have another blood test right away!"

I had the blood test and went home. A day later, Jeannie was called in to discuss my situation with the MD alone. I can only presume that this was when Jeannie asked what my chances of survival were! On returning home Jeannie said I was to get ready to go by ambulance to hospital immediately.

"Your haemoglobin count is down and you are bleeding internally, possibly bowel cancer! That is what the doctor told me," she said, soberly.

Jeannie's stress level had never been higher. I discovered later that the doctor had told Jeannie that my chances of surviving bowel cancer were "about 30% survival rate."

Jeannie packed a small bag of my clothing and toilet gear and waved goodbye from our front deck.

I was duly taken by ambulance to the hospital and arrived at about 6 p.m. There had been a delay in waiting for my mainland ambulance being diverted because of a stabbing in the area. The doctor assigned to me, was Dr. Neil Lutton. This was a pleasant surprise, as he was a close friend of the melanoma surgeon I had had months before, Dr. Chris Allen.

"You are scheduled to have two blood transfusions; the first of which will be of two and a half hours duration and the next is scheduled for the following day. That process will be of four and a-half hours' duration. You comfortable with that news?" asked Dr. Lutton.

"What's to be will be," I replied, trying to sound confident.

"Following that procedure there will be an endoscopy and colonoscopy. It is a process whereby a small camera will be inserted into your bowel to examine what exactly is going on. You will be sedated, of course, and won't feel a thing," the doctor explained.

This procedure was duly carried out within the week. Then the doctor returned and explained what they had found.

"I am bound to have to tell you that you have melanoma bowel cancer. A cell must have escaped sometime during the last procedure when you were in hospital some months ago. However, we can use the keyhole surgery procedure, which is inserted in a half-inch hole in your abdomen. The tumour will be slid into a bag to make sure no bits and pieces escape and then the whole thing is extracted through the area near your belly-button. The scar should be about four inches long. However, there is a chance that you may have to wear a bag for a short period, but it depends on what happens during the operation. Do you have any questions?"

I did have several questions to which the doctor was patient with me and answered them all. It is understandable for any one undergoing surgery to know as much as possible about the procedure and chance of survival. Well, I thought so!

The previous late afternoon, before surgery, I was given three one-litre jugs of a mixture designed to clear my whole bowel system. The drinking of the last litre was a definite challenge. Then after an hour or so I was continuously backwards and forwards on the toilet. The longest period was an hour and a half. It was not a pleasant experience. However, the morning came with me having only two hours' sleep during the whole night.

The anaesthetist was ready for me at 6.30 a.m. He was cheerful; I was mentally numb. It was not too long before he gave me an injection to steady my nerves. Then I don't recall anything specific.

I was wheeled back into my ward and left to regain consciousness. The doctor came to see me later that same day. He explained that I didn't have to have a bag attached, after all. I remember breathing a big sigh of relief. The doctor also told me that the operation was a success and that there were no further signs of cancer anywhere in the bowel area where the cancer had been.

Recovery was very painful as I experienced a great deal of wind, which as it moved through the bowel, gave off a series of painful movements. I was given endone medication for the pain, which helped to a limited degree. I was put on a more or less a liquid diet as I was not permitted to eat any solids until the bowel which had been stitched together, was strong enough to pass a motion. This was to be several weeks away.

Sleep is a commodity dosed out in small proportions in hospital. There is always some reason for waking a patient: blood pressure, blood tests, diabetes' test and taking one's temperature all add up to reduced sleep!

Jeannie visited me with a friend from the island, but Jeannie was very quiet the whole time and I knew there was something wrong. I put it done to stress. Jeannie came only one more time and even then she was quieter than usual. Once again, I put it down to a high degree of stress.

Eventually, I had two CT scans taken and when the results were known I had a visit from one of the oncologists, who asked me unusual questions.

"There seems to be something mysterious going on! Your previous CT scans of July 15, 2010, showed you were more or less riddled with cancerous tumours and now these latest CT scans show definite significant changes. Many of the tumours no longer exist, while two others have shrunken remarkably so as to be insignificant! What on earth have you been taking? You have certainly caused a stir among the oncology staff!"

His eyes widened even further when I finished giving my answer.

"Was there anything else?" he asked.

"Yes! But it is too involved to explain more fully at this point in time," I replied.

"That's very interesting! You know, we are trained to follow a certain procedure where it concerns cancer. But, recently, I've been reading about some alternative treatments. And this is the first time that I have met a patient who has actually taken an alternative treatment . . . and survived! I am quite impressed, as are some others! You are being regarded as a miracle around here!" he said, as he walked off.

Here, then, are the results of my CT scans:

Tuesday, 06 December, 2011.
CT ABDOMEN AND PELVIS
Clinical history: Metastatic melanoma. Anaemia. Blood loss.
Findings: Direct comparison is made to CT scan of 15 July 2010. Compared to that examination there has been significant improvement. No definite metastases now seen in the lower lungs on either side. The lungs have not been scanned

in their entirety but previous CT scan showed metastatic deposits in both lower lungs which are now largely resolved. Examination of the liver is compromised by the inability to give contrast. Suspicion of a very small lesion, inferiorly in segment 6 of the liver diameter 18mm much smaller than on previous CT scan. No other focal liver pathology. Spleen, pancreas and upper epigastric structures are normal. No suspicious para aortic or retroperitoneal lymph node enlargement. Adrenals and kidneys are normal. Faecal loading of the large bowel. Normal bladder outline. Right inguinal hernia containing fat and omentum. No evidence to confirm lytic or sclerotic bony metastatic disease.

Conclusion: There has been apparent substantial improvement compared to CT scan of July 2010. Although the lungs have not been scanned in their entirety there is no definite evidence of metastatic disease through the lower lungs on today's CT scan. Examination of the abdomen is compromised by the inability to give contrast. Small low density lesion seen inferiorly in segment 6 of the liver less than 2cm in diameter is substantially smaller than on previous CT scan. There is elsewhere no evidence of metastatic disease through the abdomen or pelvis. Indirect inguinal hernia, containing fat and omentum. Faecal loading of large bowel. No cause identified for the anaemia or PR blood loss. No further evidence to confirm metastatic disease.

Dr. Fergus Legh.

RESULT OF CT CHEST:
Tuesday, 06 December, 2011.

History: Metastatic melanoma to lungs and liver, progress.
Findings: Non contrast examination performed. The prior examination performed at Redland's on 15/07/2010 could not be obtained for direct comparison.

There is a very small subpleural nodule inferiorly in the right middle lobe at its anterior aspect. This measures 4mm in diameter. No other lung lesion is identified. Specifically, no cluster of nodules is identified in the left lower lobe surrounding the left lower lobe bronchi, as described on the report of the study of July 2010. Elsewhere the lungs are clear, except for a small anterior pleural based density in the lingual, 5mm in maximum diameter. This is low attenuation and is unlikely to be clinically significant.

There is no pleural thickening or effusion. The axillae are clear. No lymphadenopathy is present in the mediastinum and the hilar complexes appear normal. No destructive bony lesion is identified on bone window reviews.

Conclusion: There is no convincing evidence of metastatic melanoma within the chest. There is a small subpleural nodule anteriorly in the right middle lobe, 4mm in diameter, and this could be a granuloma or residue of a mestastasis. The examination of July 2010 described a 16mm nodule in this region. The previously described nodules in the left lower lobe measuring up to 20mm in diameter are no longer visible. No evidence of nodal or soft tissue metastatic disease.

Dr. Gregory Slater.

The report on the BOWEL CANCER is as follows:

Clinical Notes: Left colon metastatic melanoma metastasis.

Macroscopic:

The specimen container is labelled "Left colon". The specimen consists of a segment of large intestine that measures 90mm in length with an internal circumference of 86mm. One end resection margin is inked blue, the opposite ends is inked black. On the muscosal surface is an ulcerated, solid polypoid that measures 45 x 25 x 30mm. This is located adjacent to black tattoo pigment. This lesion is 30mm and 5mm from the end resection margins. The cut surface of the tumour is tan and necrotic. The tumour appears confined by the muscularis externa.

Numerous small lymph nodes are identified within the underlying adipose tissue. Some of these lymph nodes contain black pigment. Blocking Details: 1A and resection margin; 1B-1E rep sections tumour; 1F tattooed; 1G multiple lymph nodes; 1H multiple lymph nodes.

Microscopic:

Sections show an ulcerated malignant neoplasm of polygonal cells. Although no cytoplasmic pigmentation is seen, the cytological appearances are consistent with malignant melanoma. The tumour appears confined to the macosa and submucosa. The bowel resection margins are clear of tumour. There is no evidence of malignancy in eight (8) lymph nodes.

Summary:

LEFT COLON

—METASTATIC MALIGNANT MELANOMA

—NO LYMPH NODE INVOLVEMENT

—MARGINS CLEAR

Dr. Graham Adkins.

::

I was hospitalised for twenty-three days and on my release, I found there was more challenges involved.

Attempting to maintain the balance correct for passing a motion was the most difficult challenge. Each morning when I returned home, I slowly watered some garden seedlings in order to keep mobile and also to obtain fresh air and sunlight.

I knew the healing process for this operation would take its own time to heal correctly, which was estimated by my doctor to be at least eight weeks' duration. It was a very frustrating period as I was not permitted to eat a full-sized meal. I had to eat only half of a normal-sized meal in order to keep the size of the motion small.

I took extra medication for constipation for three days. This could have proved disastrous, inasmuch as a large motion could have burst the internal stitches. I drank over that period of the day four Movicol sachets. This corrected the constipation situation. But, the motion itself frightened me, as it was quite large and painful to pass. I then phoned my doctor, alarmed at what had transpired. He reassured me and told me to take double the amount of Movicol the following morning. I did as requested. Then, unfortunately, I had extreme diarrohea for the following eight days and nights! At times, it was personally embarrassing as I soiled my bed and pyjamas on several occasions, as I had no control over the flow of my motions at this stage. Jeannie cleaned up the mess without any comment. I persevered and gradually, the diarrohea decreased.

My Palliative Care nurse was contacted also during this time and she gave valuable advice. They provide a wonderful service and I, for one, am thankful for their kindness and full patient attention.

I still had severe pain in my lower abdomen caused either by passing wind or a motion. It was something that had to be endured. I tried placing a heated wheat bag over the area which lessened the pain to a small degree. It was a very slow process until quite recently, when I eventually was able to have a normal bowel movement. All through this process I was forbidden to lift anything larger than a normal tea cup, for fear of tearing the internal stitches. It was a frustrating time for a person who is usually active carrying out certain household and outside chores.

Table 1: Where Melanoma Most Likely to Spread

Organ	Likelihood of Spreading to Organ
Skin (other areas of the skin), subcutaneous tissue and lymph nodes	50-75%
Lungs and area between the lungs	70-87%
Liver	54-77%
Brain	36-54%
Bone	23-49%
Gastrointestinal tract	26-58%
Heart	40-45%
Pancreas	38-53%
Adrenal glands	36-54%
Kidneys	35-48%
Thyroid	25-39%

Source: Meyers ML, Balch CM. "Diagnosis and Treatment of Metastatic Melanoma." Cutaneous Melanoma. Balch CM, Houghton AN, Sober AJ, Soong S-J (Eds): St. Louis: Quality Medical Publishing, Inc. 1998:329.

8

Confronting My Melanoma Cancer

There is no doubt that our mental abilities are extremely powerful. Cognitive behaviour therapy, for instance, is claimed to be a very effective treatment for anxiety and depression and is a tool for analysing a patient being able to judge and reason effectively. But when you have only six months to live and you are on your own with only your thoughts to guide you, what thoughts register in your mind? If you are honest with yourself, it is likely to be "I am going to die! That is what is really going to happen to me!"

To think that we can cure ourselves of cancer simply through spiritual means, or positive thinking, is said to be dangerous and delusional. This, of course, is only an opinion and therefore, incorrect thinking and is usually stated by people who have no idea of what it is like to hear those condemning words: "You have stage IV cancer and we can no longer do anything for you!"

Turning to religion or matters spiritual in situations such as these can, and does, bring comfort and even encourages one to continue on, no matter what. To state that it is totally delusional and dangerous thinking . . . well, that person is entitled to their wrong opinion!

This is not to say that spirituality does not help people cope with cancer. The American Cancer Society says: "An analysis of forty-three studies on people with advanced cancer noted that those who reported spiritual well-being were able to cope more effectively with terminal illnesses and actually find meaning in their experience."

As for myself, treatments such as Reiki healing, energy healing, drinking many healthy concoctions and simple down-to-earth praying all gave me comfort and a sense of inner peace and, I truly feel, they all added something to my body's healing process—the immune system. Of course, I can prove nothing to substantiate such a claim. Nevertheless, nobody else can prove anything contra wise either!

Surely then, the key is to use spirituality and positive thinking, not to "order" good health as if it is on a take-away menu, but to give one the strength of character to cope with their illness to add to the offered alternative treatment. Comforting words or gestures are always beneficial to any sufferer no matter what the disease or illness and, no matter what the experts say!

The diagnostic strips that signalled the level of acidity in my body, along with bicarbonate of soda and blackstrap molasses, certainly was a piece of advice, which I would never have learned about if it hadn't been for these people: Jeannie, in knowing Vernon Johnston, and the Internet and Curtis John Mitchell. It was Vernon's courage, success and freedom from cancer that inspired me to follow his alternative treatment. But, I also added other ingredients, which I considered beneficial to my overall well-being. This led Jeannie and I to change our daily diet to one of 80 per cent alkalinity and 20 per cent acidic. It was almost like being a vegetarian, but not quite!

The most therapeutic supplemental way to add minerals to the body in the long-term is to use live products that have not been heated and also contain enzymes, anti-oxidants and a full range of vitamins and other phytonutrients. The two most obvious ones are Barley Grass Juice Powder or wheat grass. (Barley grass juice powder is enzyme rich without heat treatment is available as a supplement) and cold temperature dried sea weed, (available as a supplement such as Sea-greens). Barley grass juice powder should ideally be taken in quantity, e.g. one dessertspoon blended in cold juice or water, once or preferably, twice daily.

I also cannot stress enough the need for breathing in of fresh air for at least three-quarters of an hour every day! Cancer cannot live in a highly oxygenated area.

I am not attempting to entice, or force anyone to follow me in my treatment against cancer. I am only telling my true story! If it suits the reader to take up that challenge, then, more power to you! I allow the results to speak for themselves, even to the extent that some members of the medical profession have taken a keen interest in that alternative treatment and more importantly, the convincing truth of their own technology, the CT scans! They are forced to believe their own equipment!

Take care . . . you are not alone, after all!

9

A Private, Early-Hours Discussion

It was late at night as I lay awake in the hospital ward. Suddenly, I was approached by an oncologist who had been engaged to work at the hospital from Africa.

He looked at me and smiled, then softly said:

"I wonder if I may have a private word or two with you about the result of your CT scans?"

"Yes, of course! What do you want to know?" I asked.

"My medical training does not allow for alternative treatments for cancer because so often it is unproven. However, I have come across so many alternative treatments that are having excellent results. This, to my mind, cannot be dismissed lightly. Therefore, could you explain to me what you did to get these remarkable results, showing there are no signs of cancer now in either your neck area, both lungs and your liver? This is a truly outstanding result!"

I went on to explain the ingredients I took.

"I understand! Very interesting! Would you like to continue this talk later on?" the oncologist asked. "I am more than interested!"

I saw him again when he was accompanied by a team of oncologists on three more occasions. He smiled at me on each occasion, but never uttered a word. I never got to talk to him again.

I know that other oncologists in that hospital were interested in what I took and what I did to rid myself of cancer, but their professionalism wouldn't allow them to venture into asking questions about the world of alternative treatments!

::

Being informed could save your life!

The winds of change are certainly blowing across this world of ours and, in more ways than one! More than thirty presenters, leading practitioners in the field of holistic cancer treatments, Nutritionists, Naturopaths, Scientists, Health Advocates, Psychologists are all willing to share their knowledge on how to prevent and reverse cancer. They share their knowledge on YouTube, http:www.cancer is curablenow.tv.

This film gives you insights about our present health system and the undeniable mistakes in treating cancer as well as a comprehensive holistic healing approach to cancer never seen before. "Cancer is Curable Now" informs about all options people have for you and your family's health in curing, treating or preventing cancer as well as all other degenerative diseases.

I watched this film and was somewhat amazed that so many alternative treatments are available NOW! Numerous health providers, doctors, etc., give testimony to the value of these alternative treatments. The reason that the numbers of success is so amazing is that the normal traditional cures, surgery, radiation and chemotherapy rates of success still are in the same rate of success as years ago . . . three per cent success! Three per cent! When the amount of money that has been spent on cancer by the Cancer societies of the world is taken into account this is a shocking admission that orthodox medicine needs to take a real good look at some of the alternative treatments success stories!

"CANCER is Curable NOW" is a feature-length documentary, which covers all aspects of holistic cancer treatments and the main causes of cancer. Some people will be disappointed in the film, simply because you can never please everyone!

If you believe that cancer is going to kill you—it will! The power is within you to cure yourself and you better believe that! What you think is what you are, just as what you eat is what you are! What you think, therefore, is a very powerful motivational tool. Once again, positive thinking can help you overcome cancer, too.

People have been brewing conditions inside their bodies for at least decades. Yet, changing one's eating habits isn't at all easy! Nobody ever said it was, but changing your diet to an 80 per cent alkaline and 20 per cent acidic is one diet that will help in the battle against cancer. How do I know this? I followed the winds of change and now I am a survivor!

I am fortunate enough to be able to offer genuine hope to sufferers of melanoma cancer. Hope brings comfort and reassurance that you have not been given a death sentence, after being told that the orthodox practices can no longer do anything for you.

Think positive! Be positive!

10

An Acute Fear of Contracting Cancer

"I lost my mother four years ago to pancreatic cancer," said a distraught daughter. "Since then, I have lived in constant fear of the word 'cancer' and worry, endlessly, that I will get it. Over the past three years, I developed headaches and I was certainly convinced it was a brain tumour. I went for an MRI scan, which didn't reveal anything like cancer. Then I begged my family doctor to do tests on my liver and pancreatic. This was only recently, both of which turned out to be within the normal range.

"After a bad sinus infection, I requested a chest X-ray because I was convinced my bad cough was indicative of lung cancer. The X-ray was clear. Most recently again, I have become agitated about the possibility of stomach or colon cancer, as I have had diarrohea and a pain on the left-hand side when I press on my stomach.

"My husband is supportive, but I can see that he believes I am killing myself with the constant worry—I'm a nervous wreck. We have a wonderful life together and I want it to be a long one—but how can I learn to control my anxieties?"

I should like to think that the best thing to remember is that . . . you are not alone! But to many people that is not enough! In spite of all the worldwide research on cancer, its early diagnosis and advanced treatment modalities, cancer is seen as a dreaded disease that spells nothing but a death sentence. I wonder just how many people actually find themselves seriously worrying that they might get cancer?

Don't panic! When it comes to cancer, it is common knowledge that you are not alone. But it would seem to appear that in many people's minds they are all in the same boat and without a modicum of hope!

The fear of cancer, or Carcinophobia, is a very real disorder that affects those who have had the disease in the past and even those whose relatives and friends have been afflicted with it. Although it's regular incidence has reduced as compared to about twenty-five years ago, when knowledge and treatment of cancer was more limited, this social anxiety disorder continues to plague men and women around the world, with no lessening of the numbers more than worried.

Fear of any disease is a normal phenomenon. But when this fear becomes a continuous panic that interferes in a daily routine, then it's a problem. The reason for this fear usually stems from some sort of close association with cancer. The person suffering from Carcinophobia may have undergone a biopsy in the past. Sometimes, just seeing a close friend or relative suffer and/or ultimately die from cancer can instil this nagging fear. Often, people who have this disorder have seen the negative reactions of others to the disease and may have unconsciously begun to imitate them. Often, Carcinophobia can become so extreme that it may lead to Agoraphobia, which is the fear of being outside, or fear of being in a situation that you cannot get out of.

Different people show different symptoms of this disease. Some may start perspiring and feeling nauseous when confronted with the fear of cancer, while others, who have a more severe form of it, may have full-blown anxiety or panic attacks. Other symptoms include dry mouth, heart palpitations, numbness, and the feeling of being trapped. But, there is no need for instant panic!

Is there any treatment for this condition? Of course!

Cognitive Behaviour Therapy (CBT) is based on how the idea that how we think (cognition), how we feel (emotion) and how we act (behaviour) all interact together. Specifically, our thoughts determine our feelings and our behaviour. Therefore, negative thoughts can cause us distress and result in challenges. Fear of contracting cancer is a psychological problem rather than a physiological condition. Talking to friends and family is the initial step and may even be very helpful in relieving your stress and anxiety. Ignoring the negative people is a definite must! It has certainly been established that people generally fear something they don't have a great deal of knowledge about. Therefore, reading about cancer and its advanced treatment technologies could prove to be very helpful in relieving this phobia. The fact is, that modern medical science has made great advancements in the field, and cancer is no longer seen as a deadly disease, nor as a death sentence!

However, on the other hand, even more advancements have been made in the alternative treatments field, to the extent that large numbers of people are turning towards these remedies and turning away from unnecessary surgery, poisonous chemotherapy and crippling radiation!

Speaking with cancer survivors can also be very enlightening and extremely helpful. Ultimately, it is important to maintain a positive attitude towards life and not spend it worrying about things that may or may not happen to you or your loved ones. A further examination of this subject may prove beneficial, therefore, I have expanded on the issue for the sake of clarity.

An acute fear of being stricken with cancer is one of the most prominent long-term anxieties plaguing modern society. In many individuals, this fear can result in panic attacks that interfere with normal life. Hasn't cancer caused enough pain to those who already have this debilitating condition, including their grieving friends and relatives? It is a real tragedy that, in addition to the devastating effects of the condition itself, cancer must cause this second-order anxiety among people who don't even have cancer!

A person's ability to make rational decisions regarding cancer of whatever description—terminal or otherwise—is somewhat confused by an inner feeling that there are too many causes of cancer . . . and no easy, quick cures! Questions, such as 'good', 'bad', 'right' and 'wrong' are whirling about the patient's stressed-out brain.

Even with the best of intentions, the scientific community has the public utterly confused regarding the causes of cancer, which only adds to an over-riding fear of cancer. Deleting the dreaded fear of dying from cancer is the first step in helping the public face some true facts!

Perhaps, the most harrowing of all is anxiety about melanoma cancer, which can destroy compassion for its actual sufferers. Someone who is obsessed with the idea of harbouring a cancerous tumour in their body will avoid visiting a suffering victim of cancer—even if that victim happens to be a family member or even a close friend. Without being consciously aware of what they are doing, those who are afraid can reject family members or friends at exactly those moments when they most need help and support. I think, perhaps, it is that some people don't know what to say to people stricken with cancer!

"Hello! How are you feeling today" would be a good start! Lying in a bed or sitting alone in a chair isn't too much fun when you are left, totally disregarded by people who once were regarded as friends. It is exceptionally hard to come to terms with such a situation. Yet, the cancer sufferer can, and does, forgive. He understands . . . up to a point! We all have our breaking point!

What does the process known as metastasis comprise? The standard answer is something like this: Metastasis is the process by which cancer cells break away from a primary tumour and enter the bloodstream or lymphatic system (the system that produces, stores, and carries the cells that fight infections). That is how cancer cells spread to other parts of the body.

When cancer cells spread and form a new tumour in a different organ, the new tumour is a metastatic tumour. The cells in the metastatic tumour come from the original tumour. This means, for example, that if breast cancer spreads to the lungs, the metastatic tumour in the lung is made up of cancerous breast cells (not the lung cells). In this case, the condition in the lungs is known as metastatic breast cancer (not lung cancer). Under a microscope, metastatic breast cancer cells generally look the same as the cancer cells in the breast.

Where does cancer spread?

Cancer cells can spread to almost any part of the body, and they frequently spread to lymph nodes (rounded masses of lymphatic tissue) near the primary tumour (regional lymph nodes). This is called lymph node involvement or regional disease. Cancer that spreads to other organs or to lymph nodes far from the primary tumour is called metastatic disease. Doctors sometimes also call this "distant disease".

The most common sites of metastasis from solid tumours are the lungs, bones, liver, and brain. Some cancers tend to spread to certain parts of the body. For example, lung cancer often metastacises to the brain or bones, and colon cancer frequently spreads to the liver. Prostate cancer tends to spread to the bones. Breast cancer commonly spreads to the bones, lungs, liver, or brain. Each of these cancers can spread to other parts of the body.

Because blood cells travel throughout the body, leukaemia, multiple myeloma, and lymphoma cells are usually not localised when the cancer is diagnosed. Tumour cells may be found in the blood, several lymph nodes, or other parts of the body such as the liver or bones. This type of spread is not referred to as metastasis.

Are there symptoms of metastatic cancer?

Certain people with metastatic cancer do not have any symptoms. Their metastases are found by X-rays and other tests performed for other reasons. When symptoms of metastatic cancer occur, the type and frequency of the symptoms will depend on the size and area of the metastasis. For example, cancer that spreads to the bones is likely to cause pain of varying levels and can lead to bone fractures. Cancer that spreads to the brain can cause a variety of symptoms, including headaches, seizures, and unsteadiness. Shortness of breath may be a sign of lung involvement. Abdominal swelling or jaundice (yellowing of the skin) can indicate that cancer has spread to the liver.

Sometimes, a person's primary cancer is only discovered after the metastatic tumour causes symptoms. For example, a man whose prostate cancer has spread to the bones in his pelvis may have lower back pain (caused by the cancer in his bones) before he experiences any symptoms from the primary tumour in his prostate. Does a doctor know if a cancer is a metastatic tumour?

To determine whether a tumour is primary or metastatic, a pathologist examines a sample of the tumour under a microscope. In general, cancer cells look like abnormal versions of cells in the tissue where the cancer began. Using specialised diagnostic tests, a pathologist is often able to tell where the cancer cells came from. Markers or antigens found in or on the cancer cells can indicate the primary site of the cancer.

Metastatic cancers may be found before or at the same time as the primary tumour, or months or years later. When a new tumour is found in a patient who has been treated for cancer in the past, it is more often a metastasis, than another primary tumour.

Is a metastatic tumour possible without primary cancer?

The answer to this question is a straightforward, NO! A metastatic tumour always starts from cancer cells in another part of the body. In most cases of this type, when a metastatic tumour is found first, the primary tumour can be found. The search for the primary tumour may involve laboratory tests, X-rays, and other procedures. However, in a small number of cases, a metastatic tumour is diagnosed but the primary tumour cannot be found, in spite of extensive tests. The pathologist knows the tumour is metastatic because the cells are not like those in the organ or tissue in which the tumour is found.

Doctors refer to the primary tumour as unknown or occult (hidden), and the patient is said to have Cancer of Unknown Primary origin (CUP). Because diagnostic techniques are constantly improving, the number of cases of CUP reported by orthodox medicine is said to be decreasing.

What treatments are used for metastatic cancer?

When cancer has already metastacised, it may be treated by the orthodox treatment with chemotherapy, radiation therapy, biological therapy, hormone therapy, surgery, cryosurgery, or a combination of these. The choice of treatment generally depends on the type of primary cancer, the size and location of the metastasis, the patient's age and general health, and the types of treatments the patient has had in the recent past. In patients with CUP, it is possible to treat the condition even though the primary tumour has not been located. The aim of the orthodox treatment may be to control the cancer, or to relieve symptoms or side effects of treatment. Chemotherapy is well-known to have horrendous side-effects, without me adding more to the list.

The supposed cure rate for cancer via surgery, radiation therapy and chemotherapy, is a mere 3% cure rate of orthodox medicine. This is not a high percentage when one considers the vast amount of moneys spent by the Cancer Societies of the world, using highly priced pharmaceuticals. No wonder, then, the public has started to question the low percentage figure of supposed success when alternative treatments are having success rates that are kept well in the dark.

The liquid version of laetrile had apparently an 80% cure rate, yet, this treatment was blocked by the Food and Drug Administration in the United States years ago! The liquid version of laetrile used actually derived from Mexico where laetrile normally is extracted from apricot seeds.

Why would the Food and Drug Administration of the United States try to block the import of a cancer treatment which was totally natural and had an 80% cure rate when used as an I.V.?[1]

During my research into alternative treatments I found that alternative cancer treatments cost far less than the main orthodox cancer treatments of surgery, chemotherapy and radiation therapy; yet, alternative cancer treatments can be far, far more effective than orthodox cancer treatment! The reader doesn't need to take my word for such a statement, as Dr. Philip E. Binzel, Jr, M.D., of U.S.A., wrote a book entitled *"Alive and Well"*. In his book he explains the reasons why the FDA was adamant in trying to not only block laetrile into America but knew it was a threat to the costly cancer treatment offered by surgery, radiation therapy and chemotherapy. Dr. Binzel was also called as a witness into a Court case regarding this issue. A Court case, I might add that was won by the alternative treatment group!

It must be said that the author of *"Alive and Well"* is no ordinary doctor. He is one of those rare people who are able to speak with an honest voice. He has rejected the comforts and rewards of conformity and has chosen instead the hard path of integrity. In order to practice medicine as his conscience dictated, he had to literally, take on the entire medical establishment. It was a total uneven battle. The establishment didn't have a chance against truth!

Dr. Binzel's motive for writing this book was almost unbelievable in today's world: he simply wanted to share his knowledge so that lives could be saved. At the end of a long and successful career, he was not seeking to attract patients. In fact, he is now officially retired. He does consult with patients and their doctors from time to time, but usually at no charge. His present role is that of pioneer and teacher.

Dr Binzel originally lived in the small town of Washington Court House, Ohio. He is a classical small-town doctor, and that's exactly the way he writes. But do not be deceived. He is at the cutting edge of medical knowledge, and there are few people from the scientific community—regardless of their impressive credentials—who are willing to debate with him a second time. His folksy style and genuine humility are refreshing, but he knows his craft exceedingly well.

The title of this book, *"Alive and Well,"* is appropriate for three reasons. First, there is the happy record of the patients who have received Dr. Binzel's care. Many of them previously had been told by their original physicians that there was no hope for survival, that their cancers were "terminal," and that they had, at best, only a few more months to live. To them, many years later, the phrase alive and well has a meaning that only those who have faced death can fully appreciate.

A second significance to the title is the fact that the use of laetrile in the treatment of cancer is also alive and well—in spite of the fact that it has not been featured in the U.S. national news media since the height of its controversy in the late 1970s. Because it has not been on the evening news, many people have assumed that the treatment had been abandoned. Nothing could be further from the truth.

Finally, there is the fact that Dr. Binzel, himself, is alive and well in the sense that he has survived an incredible barrage of attacks from the medical establishment. That, in fact, is an important one. Until one understands the political power wielded by drug-oriented medicine and how that power is used against any physician who favours nutritional therapy, it is impossible to understand why nutritional therapy is not widely available to the general public.

Dr. Binzel does not use the word "cured" in describing the condition of his patients who have returned to normal life after treatment. That is more a question of semantics than substance. It is true that, once a person has developed full-blown clinical cancer—even after all their symptoms have vanished—they will have a greater-than-normal tendency to develop cancer again. That, however, assumes they return to their original life styles and eating habits. On the other hand, if they do continue to follow the dietary regimen described in this book, they will discard that handicap.

However, the question remains—are they cured? Who cares what word is used if the patient is alive and well? In orthodox medicine, they often speak of cures, but the patients are dead! According to the death certificates, they don't die of cancer, but of heart failure, lung failure, liver failure, or haemorrhage. But what caused these? They are the secondary effects of their treatments for cancer. "We got it all," is a common refrain. "I'm happy to report that we cured him of his disease—just before he died." This is not really a joke. It is the reality of orthodox cancer therapy.

The number of testimonials of patients who have turned to alternative treatments is on the rise due to the escalating success rate of alternative treatments. However, let it be known, that not all alternative treatments are bone fide, as there are some rogues who are always after a fast dollar, no matter what the circumstances to the unwary patients. But this is not to distract from those treatments that are having great success and that is what any patient wants—to be free from cancer or a lessening of their disease.

I do not claim that the alternative treatment I used is a cure for melanoma cancer. Rather, I let the results speak for themselves, including the medical profession's own CT scans results, showing that my masses of tumours were either significantly reduced or were now benign, with benign meaning non-life threatening, or had disappeared altogether! This, according to medical terminology, means that my cancer is in remission in one instance and in the other, where there are two insignificant areas, these, too, could be classified as being in remission if they have been stable for a year. I am now passed that mark! Of the two insignificant spots that have been identified, neither of which is claimed to be active. In May of 2012, I had three CT scans and a bone scan, with no signs of cancer in my body! Is that proof enough?

The cost of this particular initial alternative treatment is less than five dollars, maybe even less than that. However, the ingredients included: juicing carrots, beetroot, Barley Grass, in powder form, a celery stalk and leaves, portions of ginger, apples and a tablespoon of aloe vera juice, which are at market costs of these products. Once again, this cost will not be a deciding factor against using this treatment. The cost of a Reiki treatment or any energy-healing treatment will not break the bank either. As for prayer, who can put a cost on prayer to give one a slice of hope and encouragement and confidence to continue on? But the best news of all is in really knowing that people have already taken the first steps into taking this alternative treatment and have been successful in eliminating their melanoma cancer! Can you actually visualise the feeling in knowing that there is a melanoma treatment that doesn't cost the earth and can eliminate your cancer! There is HOPE, after all! Believe it!

Allow me to repeat what Vernon Johnston and I maintain: "No cancer survivor will tell a cancer sufferer any lies, especially, when it comes to answering questions about cancer and reliable, personally used, and now proven treatments."

(1)   Source: National Cancer Institute: Laetril/Amygdalin (PDO ®). In 1980, the U.S. Supreme Court overturned decisions by the lower courts, thereby reaffirming the FDA's position that drugs must be proven to be both safe and effective before widespread public use. As a result, the use of laetrile as a cancer therapy or as a treatment for any other medical condition is not approved in the United States, but the compound continues to be manufactured and administered as an anticancer therapy, primarily in Mexico.

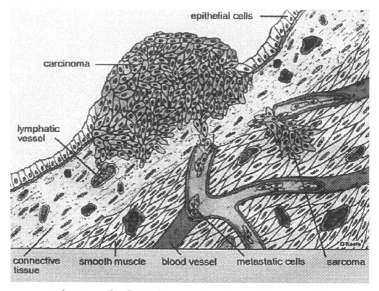

The Growth of a Melanoma Carcinoma (Cancerous).

11

"You Probably Won't Believe Me, But . . ."

Those same words above, was my introduction to Vernon Johnston, or "Vito", as he is known to many of his friends. I had sent Vernon an e-mail explaining my stage IV cancer condition and asked as to what recipe or treatment he could best advise me.

"You probably won't believe me, but, first of all, you need to find out what your body's pH level is! You do that by going to a drugstore, or the equivalent in Australia, and buy yourself some diagnostic pH strips. Then, after urinating on the strip you will find your pH level. Just using your saliva on the pH strip is not consistent, so, I found out that urinating on the strips works best.

"Whatever your pH level is, you need to get it up to pH 8.5! Yes, that is right! pH 8.5. That is the level at which cancer cannot and does not survive.

Now . . . my treatment . . . you probably still won't believe me, but . . . you take one teaspoon of bicarbonate of soda . . . yes, baking soda . . . NOT baking powder, and you mix it with one teaspoon of black strap molasses in warm water, and drink it two hours before or two hours after food, twice a day for five days at least. Then, the next morning, take another reading with your pH strip and if it isn't at the 8.5 reading, increase your bicarbonate of soda by one-half a teaspoon or one teaspoon . . . but do not increase the molasses from one teaspoon ever! Keep the pH level at 8.5 . . . that is important. Now . . . if you want any more info, go to my website, "pHkillscancer.com". This has now changed to "My Dance With Cancer". Here is what Vern has written:

The Dance Begins . . .

"Dear Son, I am coming to Hawaii. Shall I bring a tent or buy one there?"

"Dear Dad, Don't bother with a tent. I am caretaking a place and there is a vacant cabin just for you."

Well, I went to Hawaii and had one adventure after another, including camping, fire dancing, getting in between a battle between growers and rippers, announcing a couple, man and wife, at a gathering, learning Hawaiian fruits and hunting them, living in cabins, house-sitting, trip to India, two visits from my wife, getting to know my son, and much, much more.

One adventure I was not prepared for was a devastating visit to a doctor, after my return from a trip to India. Previously, I was struggling with some other health issues concerning my heart, but this one . . . this one was the 'killer'. It put me to the test.

I had passed the test in India where I made a $30.00 symbolic gesture for life by deciding to have a tooth filled instead of continuing the attitude "I am dead anyway, so why fix anything". That was huge! And I needed it to carry me through what was waiting for me. I am crying at the present moment just thinking about what happened.

A PSA test which registered 22.3 raised some huge flags, which my doctors then made appointments for a biopsy. The biopsy report indicated that I did, indeed, have prostate cancer. This called for the next step—a bone scan. The report of this scan as well as a pelvic CAT scan is where the doctors decided that I was afflicted with aggressive prostate cancer. This was March 17, 2008. The bone scan showed metastic disease at R sacrum and L. illac wing.

A second opinion from another oncologist gave me the following report: "Ancillary studies show that these are largely mentioned in the history of the present illness. The pathology confirms the presence of prostate carcinoma of high grade.

The T stage three, but without obvious invasion into the seminal vesicles on the CT scan. The radionuclide bone scan and plain films confirm the presence of skeletal metastasis in

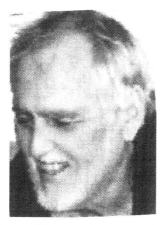

Vernon Johnston, Cancer Survivor
(Permission given to reproduce photo)

the sacrum and left illium. In addition, on review of the CT scan of the pelvis, a number of other small sclerotic leisons are noted within the pelvis. Pretreatment PSA was 22 but decreased to 5.88 after institution of finasteride and Casodex. TNM classification, T#NXM1. AJCC stage IV.

What? Stage IV? Is that what I think it says? There is no stage V! I had no idea what bone cancer was supposed to mean to me. When the first set of doctors informed me that I had prostate cancer which had spread to the bones, I didn't know if that meant my bones were going to melt away, or what!

The young doctor went on to discuss probable and improbable treatments. What he basically said is that there are none! In fact, he even mentioned that he found even more spots that the first team of doctors had missed! I was becoming used to the fact that I was a walking dead man. I was anxious to try Cesium chloride treatments but my Cesium order was lost in the mail. I started taking this on June 2nd, 2008 and stopped on 12th June, 2008. I stopped because I was scheduled for another bone scan on the 13th June, 2008. (Note: Cesium 137 is artificially produced!)

I discovered that my muscles weren't going to fall off my bones and I did get a lot of warnings about pain. Even though I was feeling better with this new information, I was still devastated. The Dance With Cancer had begun, and I don't know if I was a willing partner or not. I was just too numb! Numb as in "I felt as if my soul was sucked right out of me."

Now I am going to fast forward here a bit. You don't need to know or experience how empty I felt. So, I am jumping ahead, to the state of Oregon.

Somehow, through some miracle, my son, who lives in Las Vegas, mentioned to me something about pH and how pH affects the body. Now, this grateful information I received from my son did not get to me as I was leaving the doctor's office. It came to me after I left Hawaii.

Even though it seemed incidental at the time, having my tooth filled in India planted a seed in me that, unbeknown to me, would carry in it a desire to live.

I let the pH info I received from my son incubate for a few days before I did any pH research. The research led me to Cesium Therapy. Cesium is a mineral that, according to internet studies, likes to eat up cancer. It attacks the tumour from the inside out. And, of course, it is highly alkaline.

I was anxious to become friends with Cesium—I had nothing to lose. I do not, and did not care, what the naysayers had previously said or were saying. I wanted to do something. So, Cesium it was! But, as I mentioned previously . . . the Cesium became lost in the mail. Now what do I do? Wait for a reshipment? No! Can't do that! I'm on a roll and I need to do something quickly. The next conventional medical test is around the corner.

That is when I decided to try baking soda. It was something that I ran across on the internet that suggested that it, too, would raise my body's pH. Now, neither of these pH raising-substances indicated they would be successful in killing bone cancer. Quite the contrary! The research indicated that neither would help get rid of bone cancer. Therefore, I decided to add a twist. I added Black Strap Molasses as the carrier to the bicarbonate of soda.

I did it! I certainly did! I drank a baking soda-molasses solution. I started it on 2 June, 2008 and stopped on 12 June, 2008. I stopped, because I was scheduled for another bone scan on 13 June, 2008. They wanted to see how far the cancer had spread, or if what they were doing had slowed it down.

I need to mention here that at this "baking soda" point I was not in Hawaii. My sibling family in Oregon rallied around me and invited me to come "home" to them. They wanted to keep an eye on me; be there for me; and give me love. My real thoughts were, "I am going home . . . to die."

Luckily, the Veterans' Affairs Hospital in Portland was close by. At least, I wouldn't have to make that Hawaiian Island-to-Island jump to receive more bad news.

My son, who was in Hawaii, and whom I was having the most fun with, was totally crushed that I would leave him. He brought me to tears when he said, "Dad, stay with me! I will do whatever it takes to take care of you. I will get another job. Two, jobs, if I have to".

Believe me, that took me well over the edge. Again, this cry-baby, is crying as I write this.

But, I thought it best to go to Oregon, especially when my brother promised me that he would play Backgammon with me (I love that game). I felt I was soon to be a burden and did not want my son to be part of that. It is more complicated than that, but, I did what I thought was best at the time.

On the way to the bone scan I was hoping for hope, of any degree, no matter what! Just plain hope! I don't know why I was hoping, because all of my research indicated that once the cancer advanced into the bones you are toast! Anyway, I had the bone scan and waited for the report. It was plain hell waiting! It eventually arrived in the mail a few days later. To say that I was nervous was the understatement of the year and

I did not want to open that report at that moment. As a matter of fact, I am crying right now just thinking about it all again. I finally opened the report. It read:

NO CONVINCING EVIDENCE OF AN OSSEOUS METASTATIC PROCESS.

I bawled like a baby.

Two days later I got another report in the mail about my blood tests: PSA is now 0.1. That is zero point one!

My son, by advising me to adjusting my body's pH from acidic to alkaline as a possible way to create some ray of hope, was certainly good advice! Arm and Hammer, the manufacturers of my bicarbonate of soda had come to my rescue.

I am sure that many people are interested to know what proportions of baking soda to molasses I used. So, here goes:

I started out with one teaspoon of baking soda and one teaspoon of blackstrap molasses to one cup of water. Not warmed or heated water, just room temperature. The next day the same thing. The third day the same thing again. Fourth day the same thing again. I am feeling fine and decide to increase the dosage. I also decided to start taking notes and, finally, bought some diagnostic pH strips, so that I could measure my pH properly. My goal was to reach pH 8.0 or 8.5 pH and maintain that level for four or five days.

I read that cancer cells become dormant at pH 7 and kills them dead at pH 8 and pH 8.5.

My pH measured 7.0 pH on the fourth day when I carried out a saliva pH and 7.5 pH when I did the urine test. Then on day six: Still two teaspoons of baking soda with two teaspoons of molasses and one cup of water, twice a day. The pH measured 7.5. Was I getting any symptoms? Yes! I was feeling a little nausea. Not much, but a little queasy. My stool had a yellowish tinge to it.

Day seven. First dose was three teaspoons of baking soda, one teaspoon of molasses. I was a little nervous, therefore, a second dose. I was back to two teaspoons of the baking soda.

Day eight: two teaspoons of baking soda with two teaspoons of molasses three times a day over the day. I wanted to get the pH reading up.

Day nine: A little diarrohea, but not much. However, I was feeling a little weak, but again, not much. Later, as I thought back, it would have been a good idea to increase my potassium intake. Out of five pH readings taken over the Day Four were over 8! (7.75, 8.25, 8.5, 8.75, 8.5). I felt oxygen euphoria throughout the day. Somewhat like my body was breathing pure oxygen.

Day Ten: My headache was more persistent and I was having body sweats at night. Again the sweats duplicate Cesium symptoms. I decreased this day to a solution twice a day (two teaspoons of sodium bicarbonate and two teaspoons of molasses twice over the day. All four pH readings taken over the day were in the mid 8's.

Day Eleven: My last day before I was scheduled for the big test. The body scan was to check on the condition of my bones to see what was going on with the cancer. I dropped back to 1 ½ teaspoons of baking soda and molasses twice a day to see if it would control my headache. I had more diarrohea with slight yellow tinge. I decreased my dosage because I felt like it as I felt I was overloading. I probably would not have dropped back if I was not going to have the body scan tomorrow. The pH ranged from 8.35 to 7.25 over the day.

::

PS: Where is the Cesium? It finally showed up around 11 June, 2008. Will I take it? Yes, in a heartbeat. When? When I decide! And I decided to a few weeks later, but that is just a part of this continuing story.

Sometimes, I describe this adventure as "Being Hit by a Rainbow." You may ask, what does this have to do with being hit by a rainbow? Well, I describe anything good or miraculous, as being hit by a rainbow. My son, turning me on to adjusting the body's pH from acidic to alkaline as a possible way to create some hope was very good advice. I did not act right away on the pH factor, but within a few days I was busy on my Asus laptop, Googling away.

My sibling family bribing me out of Hawaii to come to Oregon was another rainbow hit. By the way, my brother promising to play Backgammon with me—that was a ruse. He just said that because I was not initially excited about leaving Hawaii. In fact, I was not very excited about anything. He wanted me to be close by, so he lied to me about playing Backgammon. He hates Backgammon! His goal (thank you, brother) was to get me to his house.

One of my sister's, sending me a good chunk of travel money was definitely rainbow material. Probably more like a pot of gold hitting me. She also corresponded or called me almost daily. How nice is that!

In any case, those were just a few of the getting-smacked-around-by-a-rainbow things. But the baking soda was a big one. Arm and Hammer to the rescue! I later found out that Arm and Hammer is shunned by some baking soda users because of the idea that it has aluminum in it. Wrong information! Well, at the time, I couldn't have cared less. Hey, my body is hanging on to some pretty corrupt bones. What would you do? Think about that for a second . . . that's enough for anyone!

As I later found out from research and a visit to a natural food store, aluminum is not in baking soda. It is in baking powder! The employee specialising in the vitamin and mineral department said that Bob's Red Mill Baking Powder is aluminum-free and so is, as far as she knows, all baking soda brands. I am sure there will be discussion on that!

Thank all the gods that I took notes. Larry, of Stocko fame (and a true Rainbow) on one of the Yahoo Cesium groups, drilled into me the necessity of good notes. He told me that it is for my good and for the good of others. Good for me, especially if I live! Larry, by the way, was instrumental in providing me with information. You see, he and his wife have had some of their own experiences with cancer. It is quite a story!

I met Larry while researching Cesium. He was very helpful and I was lucky to have his experience. He was definitely rainbow material and Cesium at the time was my focus. Larry sent me website after website loaded with natural cures. I cannot pretend that I read them all, but I did cruise through a few of them while waiting for my Cesium to arrive.

Well, like I mentioned earlier, the Cesium got lost in the mail. Most people would think that sucked, but not me. It was another rainbow miracle because it opened the door for baking soda to get itself busy alkalising my body.

Vernon Johnston gave me special permission to use his story in order that he and I can help others.

::

I sent Vernon an update in November 2011 and told him about my melanoma bowel cancer keyhole surgery. Here is his reply:

"Congratulations Frank . . . It must feel really good to be in charge of your Self, and to be in charge and not be angry . . . I wish you luck with the book. Thanks for letting me know. Vernon."

12

The question is . . .

What If Cancer Is Not a Disease?

While doing further research into cancer, my cognitive process suddenly asked: what if cancer is not a disease? I decided to investigate just what constituted a disease. These are my findings.

A disease is described as any disturbance or anomaly in the normal functioning of the body that probably has a specific cause and identifiable symptoms. Diseases are one of the factors that threaten people from having a properly functional life. Throughout the history of medicine, epidemics have caused the extinction of complete populations. The influenza epidemic after World War I is just one example. It has been estimated that throughout the world over seventy million people died of the influenza pandemic. In India alone, more people died of influenza than were killed all over the world during the entire First World War.

Over the last century, man has discovered many micro-organisms that cause diseases in humans and animals, and has learned how to protect himself from them, by either prevention or some kind of treatment.

An epidemic, in itself, is generally identified as a widespread disease that affects many individuals in a population. It spreads extremely rapidly through infection and simultaneously affects many people in a particular population or locality. An epidemic may also be restricted to simply one area or it may even be global. However, an outbreak of a disease is defined as being an epidemic, but, not by what pro-portion of the population it infects, but rather, by how fast the epidemic spreads.

If that information is taken as proven, then why is it that cancer is stated to be a disease when it does not appear to be infectious?

Many in the medical fraternity state that they cannot categorically agree that cancer is caused by this or that! Nevertheless, the cause of cancer does not seem to appear to be such a mystery, as science claims that there is a cause for every effect. There are many brilliant minds who have closely studied supposed causes of cancer, as well as suggesting answers to this enormous cancer challenge. Therefore, there is a desperate need for more public awareness on the actual causes of cancer so that the general public are more knowledgeable on the subject of the prevention of cancer.

The Cancer Industry

There is a definite wall of silence, almost as if it were purposeful in hiding some agenda within a special network, under common ownership and run as a single organisation with an extremely powerful authority, known to society as the cancer industry. But, what is most conspicuous is the fact that numerous sufferers from cancer are kept mystified about the clouded truths of cancer and the high technological treatments with their dramatic damaging effects on the human body. Of course, the general public have discovered by one means or another and/or seen snippets of alarming information from cancer patients themselves regarding their treatment under traditional orthodox methods. The majority of these very expensive treatments for cancer are well publicised, yet, alternative treatments which have proven to prevent and have successfully treated cancers, are discredited and their findings are never publicised by the medical authorities or the cancer industry, anywhere, or in any form, and are completely dismissed as mere quackery!

Unfortunately, the strict discipline of the orthodox medical fraternity and the cancer societies, have at some stage made the decision to withhold the whole truth about cancer, or have publicised just how little they know about it. To prevent cancer, the general public needs to understand the complete process. I suggest that the majority of people have a firm belief that cancer is a disease—but is it really a disease? There is ample evidence of documentation that proves that cancer is a symptom of many biological processes in the human body. Cancer is not such an infectious disease such as measles, mumps, poliomyelitis, or even whooping cough. Cancer has never been stated to be contagious. Nobody, to date, has ever caught cancer from someone else. Cancer is not a bacteria or a virus whose purpose is to eat the nutrients stored in our bodies.

What is the cancer industry's reasoning that they want the general public to actually believe cancer to be? The American Cancer Society states: "Although most of us think of cancer as a single disease, it is actually a family of more than one hundred different types."

What information is being revealed by this statement about cancer? It would appear to be saying that cancer is extremely complicated, overwhelming, unpredictable, and with many different types. The cancer society also calls it a disease—not just one, but over one hundred different types of diseases—a complete conglomeration of diseases. This is what the general public have been brainwashed into accepting and, somehow, believing.

Surely, society is well aware that the cancer industry profits a great deal more from cancer treatments than from cancer prevention and cancer remissions. The sickness industry makes many billions per year and cancer represents one of the biggest sources of income to the medical-drug-hospital industry. There are far more people living off cancer products than dying from it. What is wrong with that scenario?

In order to fight against cancer, the general public all over the world are asked to donate a continuum of even more money. However, is throwing millions of dollars at a vast challenge the only answer? Rationally thinking, it should not be a question of raising large sums of money for orthodox cancer research, but, indeed, for redirecting that research into directions such as proven alternative treatments.

Speaking plainly, our society is surely drug-oriented. People, everywhere, are continuously looking for a single drug or a capsule that will control their condition. Although drugs may be effective in controlling certain symptoms, no drug or capsule will ever be discovered to totally cure the many different cancers. The outward symptom of a health problem is the body's indication that its own defence system is out of kilter and is, therefore, unable to correct the adverse condition and restore health. The most effective cure for any health problem can be affected by the body's own extensive healing immune system. The human body is equipped with a marvellous healing system, superior to any healing system devised by mankind. This built-in immune system is capable of correcting any condition of ill health, if kept in the correct condition and not abused.

Wouldn't it be beneficial to all of us, if the first principle of biological medicine was to create conditions conducive to stimulate and activate the body's immune system? It will have to happen one day!

The Immune System

The traditional classification of cancer is defined by location. If a patient has cancer in the bones, it is classified as "bone cancer"; if it is in the breast, it is classified as "breast cancer"; in the blood, it is classified as "leukaemia"; in the lymphatic system, it is classified as "lymphoma." Therefore, the cancer industry identifies cancer by where it is found in the body—or in some cases, it is classified after the doctor who discovered it, or by the particular celebrity who contracted it, when it was first identified.

The renowned doctor, Arthur C. Guyton, identified in the fields of physiology and medicine, wrote a book of over one thousand pages entitled, *Medical Physiology*. In this book, he has dedicated only one single page to cancer! Dr. Guyton was obviously overly cautious about revealing what he knew about cancer! He claims, "Cancer is caused in all instances by a mutation of cellular genes."

How many of the general public have cells that are mutating? The answer is—every single person! Therefore, it is reasonable to deduce that, if every single person has cells that are mutating, then why isn't every single person dying of cancer, all at the same time?

Dr. Guyton was head of numerous degrees of research, which challenged prevailing medical cognition and, which also shaped the medical understanding of cardiac functions, hypertension, and congestive heart failure. In 1950, it is stated that Dr. Guyton carried out research proving that the cardiac output was controlled by the body tissues' need for oxygen and not by the heart itself. In addition, Dr. Guyton conducted a computer model of the circulatory system and used it to demonstrate that the kidneys provided a long-term control of the blood pressure.

Dr. Guyton further stated in his book: "Indeed, it is believed that all of us are continually forming cells that are potentially cancerous, but our immune system acts as a scavenger and nips these abnormal cells in the bud."

Unfortunately, Dr. Guyton was accidentally killed in a two-car accident in 2003, dying at the scene, whereas, his wife died a week later in hospital.

Dr. Guyton's definition of cancer is a single condition. Others of the medical fraternity differ with his opinion, stating, cancer is a naturally occurring condition of the body. It is perfectly normal and natural to have an immune system, and it is perfectly normal and natural to have a population of mutant cells. The human body has seventy-five trillion cells. It is given that in every human body there are over two hundred different types of cells. Some 230,000 cells are created every second, almost 20 billion per day. The average person is said to have approximately 1100 mutant cells daily.

Our immune systems are extremely intelligent and are, undoubtedly the most complex and critical part of the body's defence system. Yet, what causes a malfunctioning immune system? Many of the elements of our personal environment that we live in, compromise the full defence ability of the immune system. Suppressors to the immune system can be either of the physical or emotional type. Physical immune suppressors, for example, are any chemical material, which is foreign to the body and not required for a specific function. They include air and water pollutants, food chemical additives and household cleaners, pesticides, toxins, the overuse of antibiotics and other drugs and also refined sugar. Emotional immune suppressors include holding negative emotions such as fear, hate, anger, grief, anxiety, depression, resentment, frustrations, guilt, hopelessness and helplessness; debilitating stress, which overloads the nervous system, which also adds to the weakening of the immune system.

Is it possible at all to bolster the immune system? The simple answer is—yes! But, how can this be achieved? Good question! The first decision is to eliminate all the immune suppressors that can be removed. The next decision is to acquire enough immune enhancers to help with the restoration of the normal immune system. A healthy, 80 per cent alkaline and 20 per cent acidic diet, and lifestyle, is vitally important to maintaining an efficient immune system. Replace any negative emotions with positive ones. Adopt a positive, cheerful, hopeful, loving, giving and winning attitude combined with a diet primarily composed of organically grown grains, fruits and vegetables. Avoid, at all costs, wheat products, processed foods containing artificial additives. Moderate regular exercise is also very helpful and certain nutritional supplements are known to have immune enhancing effects. And, last of all, deep breathing of fresh air daily.

The immune system is designed for civil defence. It resembles an army cooperating with the natural defence and repair mechanism needed for the prevention of disease. It is composed of specialised white blood cells and a variety of organic compounds produced by the immune cells to act as regulators. The immune system has the ability to learn, identify, and then remember specific antigens, (any substance [as a toxin or enzyme] that stimulates the production of antibodies) that have been previously encountered.

Orthodox medicine battles cancers by means of drugs, surgery, radiation therapy, chemotherapy and sometimes, transplants. But, good health can only be attained by maintaining a healthy, properly functioning immune system. It is the immune system itself that fights off disease-causing microorganisms, which engineers the healing process. The immune system is certainly the main key to fighting every kind of attack on the body. Immunity is partly inherited and partly shaped by one's lifestyle. Proper nutrition plays a key role in maintaining an efficient immune system as do a number of other factors including adequate rest, emotional stability, purposeful occupation, a positive attitude, regular exercise, spiritual support, and consistent water replacement.

What do all of these components have in common with each other—Balance . . . with a capital B! When once adopting these strategies, one is able to maintain harmony in every aspect of existence—physical, mental, emotional and spiritual.

Spiritual wellness may not be something that you think much about . . . yet, its impact on one's life is unavoidable. The basis of spirituality is discovering a sense of meaningfulness in one's life and coming to know that you have a purpose to fulfil. For some people, spirituality may be equated with traditional religions such as Christianity, Hinduism or Buddhism. For others, it may mean growing in one's personal relationships with others, or through being at peace with nature.

Where are you in your spiritual life? Take a moment to reflect . . . do you feel a sense of worth, hope, purpose, commitment or peace? Do you have a positive outlook on life? Or do you experience feelings of emptiness, anxiety, hopelessness, apathy or conflict? These may be signs of spiritual poverty in your life and may be the reason for unhappiness or dissatisfaction.

Is the Immune System Frail?

The immune system will fail to heal when the strategy mentioned above is out of complete balance. What if . . . cancer just happened to be our greatest opportunity to help restore balance to aspects of our life, and furthermore, be the forerunner of severe trauma and suffering? Does that sound interesting? It means that we are always in control of our body. But, what if . . . in order to live in a human body, cancer must gain access to amounts of life-sustaining energy, and then the body may either use this inherent energy in a nourishing and self-sustaining—or in a destructive and debilitating way? Then again what if . . . in a situation we consciously, or unconsciously, choose negligence or self-abuse, over loving attention and self-respect? Our body will likely end up having to fight for its life, surely! What about the subject of spiritual health, which plays, at least, as important a role in cancer as physical and emotional reasons?

Cancer is a highly confusing and unpredictable condition. It strikes at the very happy and the very sad, the rich and the poor, the smokers and the non-smokers, the very healthy and the not so healthy. People from all backgrounds and occupations can have or attract cancer. However, if we dare look behind the mask of its physical symptoms, such as the type, appearance and behaviour of cancer cells, we find that cancer is not as coincidental or unpredictable as it seems to be.

What makes fifty per cent of conventional populations lean towards developing cancer, when the other half has little or no risk at all? Blaming one's genes is but a pitiful excuse to cover up an ignorance of the real causes. An experienced genetic researcher would smile inwardly, knowing that such a belief was void of any logic and completely unscientific[1].

Cancer has continuously been known to be a rare illness, with the exception of industrialised nations, during the past fifty years. It is said that human genes have not significantly changed for thousands of years. Why would they now suddenly change and decide to kill thousands of people? The answer is simple. Damaged or faulty genes do not kill anyone[2].

What if . . . what actually kills a cancer patient is not the tumour, but the numerous reasons behind cell mutation and tumour growth? Then, perhaps, these causes should be the focus of every cancer treatment, yet, numerous oncologists ignore them. What if . . . constant conflicts, guilt and shame, can easily paralyse the body's most basic functions, and lead to the growth of a cancerous tumour? What if . . . cancer, being the so-called physical disease, cannot mutate unless there is a strong undercurrent of emotional uneasiness and deep-seated frustration?

Some cancer patients suffer from lack of self-respect and occasionally have some "unfinished business" in their life[3]. What if . . . cancer can actually be a way of revealing the source of such inner conflict? Furthermore, cancer could, perhaps, help patients come to terms with such a conflict, and even heal it altogether. The way to take out weeds is to pull them out, along with their roots. This is how traditional orthodox medicine understands their treatment must treat cancer; otherwise, it may eventually return.

What if . . . cancer does not cause a person to become ill, but rather, it is the sickness of the person that causes the cancer? It is a medical fact that every person has cancer cells in the body all of the time. These cancer cells remain undetectable through standard tests until they have multiplied to several billion.

When doctors gleefully announce to their cancer patients that the treatments they prescribed had successfully eliminated all cancer cells, the doctors are merely referring to tests that are able to identify the detectable number of cancerous cells. Standard cancer treatments may lower the number of cancer cells to an undetectable level, nevertheless, this certainly cannot eradicate all of them. As long as the causes of tumour growth remain intact, cancer may redevelop at any time and at any rate.

Eliminating any cancer has very little to do with eliminating a group of detectable cancer cells. Treatments, such as chemotherapy and radiation therapy are certainly capable of poisoning or burning many cancer cells, but, they certainly destroy normal healthy cells in the bone marrow, gastro-intestinal tract, liver, kidneys, heart, lungs, etc., which often leads to permanent irreparable damage of entire organs and systems in the body. A real elimination of cancer should not occur at the expense of destroying other vital parts of the body.

Each year, hundreds of thousands of people who were once "successfully" treated for cancer, die from infections, heart attacks, liver failure, kidney failure and other illnesses because the orthodox cancer treatments generate a massive amount of inflammation and destruction in the organs and systems of the body. Of course, these causes of death are not being attributed to cancer. This statistical omission makes it appear that orthodox medicine is making progress in the war against cancer. However, according to the statistics of a huge number of people, they are dying from the treatment of cancer, rather than from the cancer itself. The elimination of cancer, according to orthodox medicine, is achievable only when the causes of excessive growth of cancer cells have been surgically removed, or burned, or poisoned.

The Power of the Word Cancer!

Cancer is a frightening statement, not one word, which refers to abnormal or unusual behaviour of cells in the body. However, in quite a different context, cancer is referred to as a star sign. When someone tells us that we are a "Cancer," are we going to tremble with fear of dying? It is unlikely, because our interpretation of being of the Cancer astrological sign does not imply that we have cancer, the illness. Nevertheless, if your doctor called you into his office and told you that you had cancer, you would most likely feel paralysed, numb, terrified, hopeless, or consider it as a death sentence!

The word "cancer" has the potential to play a very disturbing and precarious role. One that is capable of delivering a terrifying death sentence. Being a cancer patient begins from the very first moment you are diagnosed with cancer, although the cause of that cancer may have been there for many years, even before you began to feel unwell. Within a brief moment, the word "cancer" can turn someone's entire world upside down, inside out and every other which way as well.

Who, or what, in this world has presented this simple word with such great power that it can have command over life and death? Or does it? Could it actually be that our collective, social belief that cancer is a killer disease, in addition to the aggressive treatments that follow diagnosis, are largely responsible for the current dramatic escalation of cancer in the orthodox hemisphere? Too far-fetched, some might say! Yet, cancer can have no power or control over anyone, unless it is unconsciously allowed to grow in response to the beliefs, perceptions, attitudes, thoughts, and feelings, which are aroused because of that one word, cancer!

Would the general public be just as afraid of cancer if it knew what caused cancer or, at least, understood what its underlying purpose was? Unlikely! If the whole truth was told, the general public would most probably do everything to remove the causes and, thereby, set the preconditions for the body to heal itself.

A little knowledge (or should that be a lot ignorance) is, in fact, a dangerous thing. Almost everyone, at least in the industrialised world, knows that drinking water from a filthy source or even a polluted source can cause life-threatening diarrohea, or even leptospirosis, but still only few people realise that holding on to resentment, anger and fear, or eating fast foods, chemical additives, and artificial sweeteners, is no less dangerous than drinking polluted water; it may just take a little longer to kill a person than a tiny amoeba.

Mistaken Judgment

It is generally comprehended that if the foundation of a house is strong, the house can easily withstand external challenges, such as a storm. Cancer can show that life as a whole (physical, mental and spiritual) stands on shaky ground and is quite fragile, to say the least. It would be a sign of gardening incompetence for a gardener to water the withering leaves of a tree when he should know that the real problem is not where it appears to be, namely, on the withered leaves. By watering the roots of the plant, he naturally attends to the causative level, and consequently, the plant regenerates itself swiftly and automatically.

To the experienced gardener, the symptom of withering leaves is not a sign of a disastrous disease. The experienced gardener recognises that the dehydrated state of these leaves is but a direct consequence of withdrawn nourishment that they need in order to sustain themselves and the rest of the plant.

This example accurately describes one of the most fundamental principles controlling all life forms on earth. However adept a person may mastermind the functions of the human body through the application of orthodox medicine, this basic, highly-evolved principle of evolution cannot be suppressed or violated without paying the hefty price of side-effect-riddled suffering and pain—physically, emotionally and spiritually.

What if . . . cancer is not a killer disease? According to the definition of a disease, cancer is not a disease at all! Many people who have received a "terminal" cancer sentence and have actually defied the prognosis and turned to alternative treatments, have, against all orthodox reasoning, experienced total remission. These are termed as miracles!

What Are the Answers?

There is not one case of cancer that has not been survived by someone—regardless of how far advanced it was[4]. If even one person has succeeded in overcoming his death threat of cancer, there must be a mechanism for it, just as there is a mechanism for creating cancer. Every person on this earth has the capacity for both.

If a patient has been diagnosed with cancer, he/she may not be able to change the diagnosis, but it is certainly in their power to alter the destructive consequences that the diagnosis may have on them. The way a patient visualises the cancer and the steps taken following the diagnosis are some of the most powerful determinants of future health, or the lack of it.

The indiscriminate reference to "cancer" as being a killer disease by medical professionals has turned cancer into a condition with tragic consequences for the majority of today's cancer patients and their families. Cancer has become synonymous to extraordinary suffering, pain and death. This is true, despite the fact that 90-95 per cent of all cancers appear and disappear out of their own accord. There is not a day that passes without the body making millions of cancer cells.

Some people, under severe temporary stress make more cancer cells than usual and form clusters of cancerous cells that disappear again once they feel better. Secretions of the DNA's anti-cancer drug, Interleukin-2—a type of chemical messenger, a substance that can improve the body's response to disease, which stimulates the growth of certain disease-fighting blood cells in the immune system—drop under physical and mental duress and increase again when relaxed and happy[5]. Therefore, most cancers disappear without any form of medical intervention and without causing any real harm—thanks to a healthy immune system!

Right at this very moment, there are millions of people with cancers in their body walking around without having a clue that they have them. Also, there are millions of people who heal their cancers without even knowing it. Overall, there are many more spontaneous remissions of cancer than there are diagnosed and treated cancers.

The truth is that relatively few cancers actually become "terminal." However, once diagnosed, the vast majority of all cancers are never even given a chance to disappear on their own. They are promptly targeted with an arsenal of deadly weapons of cell destruction such as chemotherapy drugs, radiation therapy and the surgical knife. The problem with cancer patients is that, terrified by the diagnosis, they submit their bodies to all of these slash/burn/poison procedures that, more likely than not, lead them to the day of final sentencing: "We have to tell you that there is nothing more that we can do to help you." I know those words only too well, from personal experience!

The most pressing question is not how advanced or dangerous a cancer is, but what needs to be done to not end up dying from it. Why do some people travel the journey of cancer as if it were simply the flu? Are they lucky or is there some mechanism at work that triggers the healing? In other words, what if . . . there is an element that prevents the body from healing cancer naturally, or what if . . . there is a hidden element that makes cancer so dangerous—if it is dangerous at all?

The answers to these questions lie with the reply of the patient who has the cancer, and not with any degree of cruelty or progressive stage. Does the general public accept that cancer is a disease? The most probable answer will be "yes," mainly because of the given "informed" opinion that the medical industry and mass media have fed to the general public for decades. Yet, the most pressing, yet rarely asked, question remains: "Why does society consider that cancer is a disease?"

"Because I know that this dreaded cancer kills people every day." I would add another question: "How does the general public know that it is the cancer that actually kills people?" The answer would, more than likely be that most people who have cancer die, so obviously, it must be the cancer that kills them! Besides, it may be reasoned, that all of the expert medical professionals tell us so.

Although there is no scientific proof whatsoever that cancer is a disease (as opposed to a survival mechanism), most people will insist that it is a disease because this is what they were told to believe. Yet, their belief is only hearsay information based on other people's opinions. These other people heard it from someone else. Eventually, the "truth" of cancer being a disease can be traced to some doctors who expressed their subjective feelings or beliefs about what they observed and wrote about in some review articles or medical reports. Other doctors agreed with their opinion, and before long, it became a "well-established" fact that cancer is a vicious illness that somehow gets hold of people in order to kill them. However, the truth of the matter may be quite different.

Intelligence of Cancer Cells

What if . . . cancer cells are not part of a malicious disease process? When cancer cells spread (metastacise) throughout the body, it is not their intentionality to disrupt the body's vital functions, infect healthy cells and obliterate the body. Self-destruction is not the theme of any cell unless, of course, it is old and worn out and ready to be turned over and replaced. Cancer cells, like all other cells, "understand" that if the body dies, they also will die. Simply because some people assume that cancer cells are there to destroy the body, it does not mean that cancer cells have such an intention.

A cancerous tumour is neither the cause of progressive destruction nor does it actually lead to the death of the body.

There is nothing in a cancer cell that has even remotely the ability to kill anything. What eventually leads to the demise of an organ or the entire body is the wasting away of cell tissue resulting from continued deprivation of nutrients and life force. The drastic reduction or shutdown of vital nutrient supplies to the cells of an organ is not primarily a consequence of a cancerous tumour, but actually its biggest cause.

Microbes Can Live Without Oxygen

There are many types of microbes (bacteria and fungi) that are able to live in the absence of oxygen. These organisms either do not have the enzymes required to detoxify oxygen waste, or they are not able to make enough of these enzymes to be able to live at normal levels of atmospheric oxygen. These microbes are called anaerobes. They are still able to break down food molecules in the absence of oxygen, but cannot do so as efficiently as aerobes.

Although they are not able to get as much energy from their food, being an anaerobe has its advantages. Microbes that do not require oxygen are able to live in places where aerobes cannot survive, such as the human gut, and many other places where oxygen is in low supply. For pathogenic microbes (those that cause disease), this ability is a huge advantage, allowing anaerobic pathogens to cause disease in areas of the body that are not exposed to oxygen.

By definition, a cancer cell is a normal, healthy cell that has undergone genetic mutation to the point that it can live in an anaerobic surrounding (an environment where oxygen is not available). In other words, what if . . . somehow, a group of cells are deprived of vital oxygen (their primary source of energy), some of them will die, but others will manage to alter their genetic software program and mutate in a most ingenious way: the cells will be able to live without oxygen and derive some of their energy needs from such things as cellular metabolic waste products?

If that were the situation, then it may be a great deal easier to understand the cancer cells' phenomenon when comparing it with the behaviour of common micro-organisms. Bacteria, for example, are divided into two main groups, aerobic and anaerobic, meaning, those that need to use oxygen and those that can live without it. This is important to understand since the human body has more bacteria than the body has cells. Aerobic bacteria thrive in an oxygenated environment. They are responsible for helping the body with the digestion of food and manufacturing of important nutrients, such as B-vitamins. Anaerobic bacteria, on the other hand, can appear and thrive in an environment where oxygen does not reach. They break down waste materials, toxic deposits and dead, worn out cells[6].

The body sees the cancer as being such an important defence mechanism that it even causes the growth of new blood vessels to guarantee the much-needed supply of glucose and, therefore, survival and spreading of the cancer cells? What if . . . the body knows that cancer cells do not cause but, rather, prevent death, at least, until the wasting away of an organ leads to the demise of the entire organism? Therefore, if the trigger mechanisms for cancer are properly taken care of, such an outcome can be avoided[7].

The fact that our immune system protects the body against cancer seems to be only partially true. On the one hand, the immune system readily destroys the millions of cancer cells that a healthy human body produces as part of the daily turnover of thirty billion cells. On the other hand, the immune system takes no action to eradicate cancer cells that develop in response to a build-up of toxins, congestion and emotional stress. Why, especially, if cancer is composed of the bad cells that they are supposed to be?

Cancers and all other tissues in the body are loaded with cancer-killing white cells, such as T-cells. In the case of kidney cancer, and melanomas, for example, white cells make up fifty per cent of the mass of the cancers. Since these T-cells easily recognise foreign or mutated cell tissue such as cancer cells, it would be expected that these immune cells would attack cancer cells immediately.

The immune system allows cancer cells to recruit it to actually increase and spread the cancer to other parts of the body? Cancer cells produce specific proteins that reprogram the immune cells to leave them alone and help them to grow[8].

Surely, the immune system wouldn't want to cooperate with any cancer cells to make more or larger tumours, would it? Maybe, cancer is more devious than ever imagined? Then, why doesn't the immune system eradicate cancer cells that develop in response to a build-up of toxins, congestion and emotional stress?

One thing is for certain . . . maybe, cancer cells are more intelligent than we give them credit for!

References:

(1) Andreas Moritz "Cancer is Not a Disease. It's a Survival Mechanism."
(2) Ibid.
(3) Ibid.
(4) Ibid.
(5) Ibid.
(6) Ibid.
(7) Ibid.
(8) Ibid.

13

"Ideal pH" Different From What Others Teach?

There are numerous examples coming to the fore about the success rate for alternative treatments every day. I should know . . . I am a recent cancer survivor! After being told that the medical profession can no longer do anything for you . . . you feel confused and your brain goes numb! But the truth is that you are left to your own devices. But no longer!

What you do about that should really be your concern. However, it concerns me as well and that is one reason why I wrote this book.

The typical cancer patient today, who seeks out alternative treatments usually has had quite extensive chemotherapy and radiation (and may still be using them) and has probably had some major surgery.

Their cancer has already spread significantly, the cancer is spreading quickly, their immune system has been destroyed for several reasons, they have large amounts of lactic acid in their bloodstream, their liver and bloodstream are full of microbes, their digestive tract can barely extract nutrients from any food because of damage by chemotherapy, etcetera.

I was an advanced cancer patient with one foot in the grave and the other on a banana skin!

The fact that 95% of U.S. cancer patients who visit the Cancer Tutor website have already had extensive orthodox cancer treatments. The Cancer Tutor website is the Natural

Cancer Treatment for Advanced Cancer Patients run by R. Webster Kehr, the Independent Cancer Research Foundation Inc. Many of these people have spent their life-savings paying their "health" insurance company and have no money remaining for alternative cancer treatments; or you may prefer the name, complementary medicine. This is why there is a need for alternative cancer treatments, which are proven effective, yet, at the same time, inexpensive.

Some of the treatments mentioned here cost less than $100, yet they are very effective! This website contains information about alternative cancer treatments, which are among the least expensive on earth. Actually, many of them are free. One costs about $3.00.

Even though these cancer treatments are inexpensive, do not think for one moment that they are not effective. Because they are! These treatments are a significant part of the vast arsenal of cancer treatments every cancer patient should be familiar with. For example, you will note in studying this website that many of the most potent cancer treatments contain at least one of these four items:

1. Cesium (e.g. cesium chloride), (highly alkaline).
2. Baking Soda, Sodium Bicarbonate or $NaHCO_3$ (highly alkaline).
3. Calcium (e.g. coral calcium) (highly alkaline).
4. Vitamin C.

But, have you heard of Dr. Carey Reams and his RBTI Analysis, which stands for Ream's Biological Theory of Ionisation? RBTI Analysis is a tool, which trained practitioners use to measure the residues and components in samples of urine and saliva. This enables specialists to see where your body is out of balance and how to design a program to help you achieve optimal health.

After considerable thought, I came to the conclusion that the cause and the treatment for most, if not all disease, was found in 1976 by Dr. Carey Reams. He concluded that, as in agriculture, the soil determines the disease, inasmuch that a bad soil yields unhealthy vegetables, which are prone to parasites, to rot, fungi, etc. Inside a human body, the same applies. When the soil, i.e. the blood pH, the mineral and vitamin status is bad, the blood and tissue become a place where microbes transform into pathogenic microbes (viri, bacteria, moulds, fungi, yeasts) and start to destroy the host. At the same time, they try to create the perfect habitat by excreting acids that make the soil even worse, so these microbes can thrive inside the body.

Ream's Biological Theory of Ionisation has been used in clinical practice for over 50 years and has helped many thousands of patients. It has been named after Dr. Carey Reams, the scientist, who through extensive laboratory testing and mathematics came up with these trained practitioners to realise the formula for perfect health.

It is reported that a similar system is used in naturally based agricultural practices to enhance crop yields with healthier fruit, vegetables and even livestock. This system has been developed and refined over many years and it has been successfully used to assist in the health of babies, children, teenagers, adults and senior citizens. The residues and components of urine have been used since ancient times and are still in use today in medical science to test for imbalances in the human body. Any variations that arise from perfect balance, indicate how well the person has been chewing, digesting and processing their food and, therefore, what energy any patient may have available from that food.

The ideal pH, according to Dr. Carey Reams' life-time of work in agriculture, animal and human health, is 6.40 pH. There is no doubt, based on experience in agriculture and human health with Dr. Reams' work, that he was the only one aware of who thoroughly understood the how, where and whys of pH as connected to the frequencies of biologic life.

"There are other medical practitioners, who propound higher pH readings as 'ideal,' however, they do not, apparently, fully understand body chemistry. They typically arrive at their misunderstandings by looking at the pH of blood and then assume their conclusions," said Dr. Reams. "Blood pH has to maintain a very narrow margin between 7.35 and 7.45 in order to maintain life. Blood pH is not the same as the pH of extracellular fluids and this is where those assumptions fall apart.

In addition, those who teach a higher pH as "ideal" do not understand the "real" aspects that pH represents in body chemistry.

There are some misconceptions about bicarbonate of soda that need to be rectified. Firstly, there is NO aluminium in bicarbonate of soda, whatsoever. The aluminium will be found in Baking Powder, NOT bicarbonate of soda! Another misconception is that survivors of cancer do NOT take Bicarbonate of Soda and blackstrap molasses on an empty stomach and then go for a five-mile run! This can have serious consequences. *Do not even attempt it!*

14

Some Answers Are Least Expected!

No doubt it is well known that we are what we eat, but really, we are what we absorb. Our bodies depend on the nutrients we feed it to survive, regenerate and replicate on a cellular level. Every 90 to 120 days our bones, skin and blood completely regenerate. Most of the processed foods we eat are full of food "stuffs", empty calories and preservatives, which cause cellular starvation and cravings, leading to obsessive snacking and weight gain.

I would like to suggest to everyone who either has cancer or wants to prevent it, to open up to the reality that you are a whole person and diet alone is not the way to health.

When I was first diagnosed with cancer, the shock of the diagnosis instigated an initial thought, which was to do something quickly! Like NOW! It took me only a moment to comprehend what I had been told.

Cancer is a late-stage warning sign that something is definitely wrong with the entire system—definitely not just the physical body! However, it is not too late to possibly restore the system, but It cannot be accomplished by diet and exercise alone! The original discovery that cancer cannot survive proper levels of oxygen in cells, and conversely thrives in low oxygen conditions, was made back in the 1930's in Germany by a Dr. Siegel. This piece of information got me to thinking as to why Dr. Siegel's discovery has never been fully explored. Well, measures are now leading to more open doorways regarding the proper levels of oxygen in our cells.

I was asked to explain the connection between tissue pH and oxygenation. It was not because I was in any way connected to any medical association or founding institution. It was simply that I had asked for some advice pertaining to melanoma cancer and bicarbonate of soda and blackstrap molasses, which I had used to eradicate my body of melanoma cancer.

The answer was provided by a Regenerative Nutrition, a Natural Health spokesman: "A new cancer paradigm; one that is based on an understanding that cancer is ultimately caused by multiple interacting factors that combine to invite primary yeast and fungi infections, to destroy your life."

Cancer is a prime example of how heavy metal toxicity, free radical damage, pathogen infection, mineral and vitamin deficiencies, inflammation, mitochondria dysfunction, (causing oxygen deficiency) immune system depression, and oxidative stress, all come together into an end stage life threatening condition. Cancer treatment can be approached in many ways but the best way would be to address all these problems simultaneously.

Once you have undertaken a course of intensive bicarbonate of soda treatment it is sensible to keep an eye on your body's pH level. It is probably a very good practice to keep taking molasses on their own twice a day on a more or less permanent basis to keep up the alkaline minerals in the body, and if pH slips too low i.e. below 6.5 on a consistent basis (urine test) introduce some bicarbonate of soda again e.g. one teaspoon, twice daily, until the pH increases.

In my opinion, cancer sufferers must redouble their efforts to alkalise their bodies in the long-term with suitable diet and remedies such as Barley Grass juice powder. For long term alkalisation and well-being, all minerals are required, not just sodium bicarbonate as a means of alkalisation. Furthermore, the balance of sodium to potassium, calcium to magnesium and so on, should be fostered and maintained. A low cost way of doing this is to take one dessertspoon of organic molasses in a cup of hot water twice daily. This is very rich in minerals and has been responsible for cancer remissions as detailed in Cyril Scott's book, *Crude Black Molasses*. Adding refined sugars or refined grains to the diet (such as bread and biscuits etc., which are not 100% whole grain) is recognised as a good way in continuing to be ill.

One of the reasons for this is that these items acidify the cells. The minerals that have been removed from these foods are the elements that alkalise the body. That is why whole, especially raw, fruits move one towards health and alkalisation. A good example is the sugar cane. The sugar cane juice may be considered a whole food like a fruit juice, very rich in minerals. Sugar is produced, basically by removing the valuable minerals from sugar cane. Regular consumption of refined sugar causes mineral depletion in the body and an acid state. On the other hand, the minerals that have been left behind in the sugar-making process are super concentrated and are therefore, a good source of minerals, and tend to heal and alkalise the body. Molasses does have some remaining sugar content, but this is lower percentage wise than the original sugar cane, therefore, the concentration of alkalising minerals is more than able to balance this.

An interesting book to read is: *Take This Book to Hospital With You!* The authors are Charles B. Inlander and Ed Weiner, People's Medical Society, 1993. It is available from the People's Medical Society, 462 Walnut St., Allentown, PA 18102, U.S.A., or from Amazon.com.

This book is the ultimate consumer's guide to surviving a hospital stay, Take This Book to Hospital With You, gives the inside information that most U.S. hospital administrators would prefer that you do not know. How to avoid getting a hospital-acquired infection—one out of every ten people admitted become infected! How to change your room, your doctor, or your nurse! Which hospital departments are most likely to commit malpractice. What rights you sign away, or think you do, on a hospital consent form. How to scrutinise your bill for errors—numerous studies have found that more than 90% of the hospital bills reviewed had errors, mostly in favour of the hospital.

15

Communicating and Cancer Survival

Communicating with your spouse/partner about how cancer has affected you can be extremely difficult. Non-communicating is far worse! Even strong relationships can become strained under the pressure of managing a complex illness. Taking the steps to improve your communication skills can help you to feel more supported and understood.

Why is it important for survivors to communicate well with their partners?

A spouse or partner can be a primary source of support to a cancer survivor. However, if communication begins to break down, it can be stressful and result in low levels of support for both. While the cancer journey can be emotionally challenging for survivors, it can also be hard on loved ones, too. In some cases, a partner may experience more emotional distress than the survivor.

Both survivors and their partners may have strong emotions such as fear, anger and guilt. Stress is also common. A decline in the physical or emotional status of either may create a "cycle of distress" for the couple. If this happens, one person's distress also affects the other. High levels of emotional distress can strain the relationship. Good communication may be the most effective strategy for breaking this cycle. It may also improve the quality of life for both. Here are a few guidelines that may help[1] :

- Practice active listening. Active listening is when you concentrate on understanding what your partner is saying, rather than thinking about what to say next. Restate what your partner said in your own words and then ask for feedback to make sure you understand your partner's point of view.
- Don't assume you know what your partner is thinking or feeling or what your partner will say next. Ask questions if something may be unclear.
- Use "I" statements to describe your feelings rather than blaming one's partner. For example, "I felt sad when you didn't want to go to the movies with me," instead of: "You never want go anywhere with me!"
- Be specific. Avoid unclear words (for example, "hurt" could mean either sad or disappointed) and talk about specific events rather than generalisations (for example, "Please don't leave your socks on the floor," rather than "You're so messy!").
- Avoid criticism, sarcasm, name-calling, and insults. Please! Do not yell!
- Go slowly. Take some time to sort out what you want to say and to find the words you want to use. Don't pressure your partner into responding too quickly.
- Take turns talking and don't interrupt each other.
- Focus on one topic at a time. Avoid bringing up other topics or old arguments.
- If you become angry or upset, take a deep breath and consider taking a break until you feel calmer.
- Don't expect to resolve difficult topics in one conversation. Agree to continue talking at another time.

Here are some guidelines that may help you talk with your spouse or partner about cancer, how it makes you feel, and how it affects you and your relationship. Because cancer changes the lives of each person in a relationship, both partners need to talk about how cancer affects them[2].

Talk openly about treatment options and work together to make treatment decisions. Whenever possible, attend doctors' appointments together so you have shared information.

- Choose times to discuss things when you are both free from distractions and not rushed. Some couples find that scheduling a daily time to sit down and talk works well.
- You don't always have to talk about cancer. Remember to talk about normal things as well—just talking, helps couples feel closer.
- If you have something especially difficult to discuss, it may help to practice what you want to say or write notes for yourself.
- Because you and your partner probably have different ways of coping with stress, you may have differing needs for your conversations. One partner may view cancer as a problem to be solved, while the other needs emotional support and validation. Discuss fully these differences and understand that both points of view have value.
- Talk honestly and openly about your feelings, both positive and negative. Emotions such as anger, fear, frustration, and resentment are normal reactions to a diagnosis of cancer. Couples often don't discuss these emotions for fear of upsetting the other partner or because they feel guilty for having negative thoughts. Hiding one's feelings creates distance between partners and prevents them from supporting and comforting each other.
- You and your partner will not always feel the same way—you may be more apprehensive while your partner may be more hopeful. Talk about these differences and respect your partner's feelings.
- Tell your partner how you are really feeling physically and emotionally. This sharing helps your partner understand your challenges and gives an opportunity for your partner to support you.

- Tell your partner often about the specific types of support and encouragement that you need. One day you may need encouragement to get out of the house, while another day you may need some quiet time alone.
- Humour may help you and your partner cope, so don't be afraid to laugh.

Good communication skills can help survivors and their partners to:

- Receive and offer emotional support.
- Get help making decisions.
- Share advice and encouragement.
- Learn new ways of handling stressful situations.
- Clarify misunderstandings.
- Learn new coping strategies.
- Plan for the future, such as family, employment and financial decisions.
- Important issues that partners may need to discuss together include: Ways to solve problems with changing roles and responsibilities in the relationship.
- Instructions and preferences for decisions about health care and financial matters.
- Concerns about changes to sexual relations and expressions of intimacy.
- Challenges adjusting to the cancer experience.
- How to maintain the quality of the relationship.

The cancer experience can be a time that enriches and strengthens the relationship. A partner can play a large role in shaping the emotional experience of the survivor to the experiences of cancer and life after treatment. Research shows that survivors who feel they have support from their partners are more likely to focus on the positive aspects of their cancer journey. This can improve their quality of life.

Why is it sometimes difficult for survivors to communicate with their partners? There may be a number of reasons why it can be difficult for survivors to communicate with their partners. A partner's negative response to the survivor's discussions may discourage open communication.

Research shows that a survivor is negatively affected if his or her partner uses criticism, withdrawal or acts uncomfortable, especially when the survivor talks about the cancer experience. This may cause the survivor to use fewer healthy and effective coping strategies. Emotional problems can result and a cycle of distress may occur in the relationship.

Negative responses from partners that may make communication difficult include:

- The partner does not want to talk about what the survivor is experiencing because it is far too upsetting.
- The partner feels over-protective and tries to prevent the survivor from doing things.
- The partner wants the survivor to get back to normal and try to forget that the cancer experience happened.

The cancer journey may require that couples communicate about topics that they normally would not talk about. Issues, such as the side effects or after-effects of cancer and treatment, may be difficult to discuss. For example, some survivors experience incontinence, sexual or fertility problems or changes in self-esteem and body image. These may be very hard for some people to talk about openly.

The cancer journey may involve long-lasting complications, such as fatigue and chronic pain, and it may be difficult for partners to fully comprehend. This is very true when the survivor is in remission, or looks healthy. The partner may want the survivor to move on and return to life the way it was before the cancer.

Sensitive issues that may be difficult to discuss include:

- Living with uncertainty.
- Stress.
- Feelings of guilt.
- Financial difficulties.
- Dealing with fear of recurrence.
- Changes in outlook on life and death.
- Other health and physical problems.
- Losses of all kinds including job, friends, abilities.
- Changing roles and responsibilities.
- New compromises that need to be made.
- Feeling overwhelmed.
- Anger.
- Survivors may feel guilty trying to discuss certain topics with their partners.

It can be quite difficult for survivors to ask others for help—war veterans, especially so. This is particularly true if the survivor has always been the one to help others. Some may continue to try to do tasks that have become too emotionally or physically challenging.

Some survivors are worried about the stress on their partners. They may feel guilty about asking partners to take on new roles and responsibilities. They may be concerned that a partner is as distressed (or more) than the survivor. A survivor may try to protect his or her partner by not sharing information. Important discussions about certain topics, such as health care directives and financial matters, may be avoided in an effort not to upset the partner.

Survivors and partners may have totally different priorities. Cancer survivors and their partners may find that some things that were important to them before treatment are no longer as important. There may be a change in the way they view life. Some decide to change jobs or other relationships in their lives.

Sometimes, both partners and survivors can easily understand the change in priorities and be comfortable with them.

Other times, one of them might not understand why these changes are happening or may not agree with them. This can feel threatening to any relationship.

How can survivors learn to communicate well with their partners? Couples sharing the cancer journey can learn new and effective communication strategies. Even though it can be difficult to change old habits, learning skills and developing new communication habits is possible. The key is to practice the new skills regularly. The benefit is that healthy communication can increase satisfaction in a couple's overall relationship and positively affect the quality of life for both.

Some ways to improve communication skills include:

- Being aware of your own communication patterns and behaviours.
- Understanding the communication patterns and behaviours of your partner.
- Learning and practicing effective communication skills together.
- Discuss difficult topics with your partner.

How can better communication benefit survivors and their partners? There may be many times when survivors and their partners have a hard time talking with one another. During times of stress, effective and healthy communication might be a challenge for couples. This can be especially difficult if there were already problems talking and sharing even before the cancer diagnosis.

If communication between you and your partner is not what you would like, you need to work on building skills. You may be able to do this or with the help of a licensed counsellor.

References:

(1). American Society of Clinical Oncology.
(2). Dr. Cindy L. Carmack Taylor, Ph.D., The University of Texas, M.D. Anderson Cancer Center.

16

Difference Between Blood pH and Urine pH

pH: What does it mean? pH is the abbreviation for potential hydrogen. The pH of any solution is the measure of its hydrogen concentration. The higher the pH reading, the more alkaline and oxygen rich the fluid is. The lower the pH reading, the more acidic and oxygen deprived the fluid is. The pH range is from 0 to 14, with 7.0 being neutral. Anything above 7.0 is alkaline, anything below 7.0 is considered acidic.

Human blood stays in a very narrow pH range right around (7.35-7.45). Below or above this range means symptoms and disease. If blood pH moves too much below 6.8 or above 7.8, cells stop functioning and the patient dies. The ideal pH for blood is 7.4

A healthy blood pH without cancer has acid + alkaline balance almost equal. Actually a healthy body is slightly alkaline measuring approximately 7.4. This ideal blood 7.4 pH measurement means it is just slightly more alkaline than acid.

The pH in the human digestive tract varies greatly. The pH of saliva is usually between 6.5-7.5. After we chew and swallow food it then enters the upper portion of the stomach which has a pH between 4.0-6.5. This is where "predigestion" occurs while the lower portion of the stomach is secreting hydrochloric acid (HCl) and pepsin until it reaches a pH between 1.5-4.0. After the food mixes with these juices, it then enters the duodenum (small intestine) where the pH changes to 7.0-

8.5. This is where 90% of the absorption of nutrients is taken in by the body while the waste products are passed out through the colon (pH 4.0-7.0).

If you have a health problem, most likely your body is acidic. Research shows that unless the body's pH level is slightly alkaline, the body cannot heal itself. Therefore, no matter what type of modality you choose to use to take care of your health problem, it won't be as effective until the pH level is up. If your body's pH is not balanced, you cannot effectively assimilate vitamins, minerals and food supplements. Your body's pH affects everything.

The body has to have a balanced pH like most living things on earth, or it does not function correctly. The alkaline level is very important because research has already proven that disease cannot survive in an alkaline state, and yet, they thrive in an acidic environment.

The truth is everyone has different nutrient requirements, but we all share one thing in common—we need to have alkaline blood to stay healthy.

An acidic balance will: decrease the body's ability to absorb minerals and other nutrients, decrease the energy production in the cells, decrease its ability to repair damaged cells, decrease its ability to detoxify heavy metals, make tumour cells thrive, and make it more susceptible to fatigue and illness.

An acidic pH can occur from an acid forming diet, emotional stress, toxic overload, and/or immune reactions or any process that deprives the cells of oxygen and other nutrients. The body will try to compensate for acidic pH by using alkaline minerals. If the diet does not contain enough minerals to compensate, a build-up of acids in the cells will occur.

There are two factors that are always present with cancer, no matter what else may be present. Those two factors are Acid pH and lack of oxygen. Can we manipulate those two factors that always have to be present for cancer to develop and by doing so may help reverse the cancer? If this is so, then we need to learn how to manipulate those two factors.

Cancer needs an acid and low oxygen environment to survive and flourish within. Terminal cancer patients are around one thousand times more acidic than normal healthy people. The vast majority of terminal cancer patients possess a very low body pH. Why?

In the absence of oxygen, glucose undergoes fermentation to lactic acid. This causes the pH of the cell to drop from between 7.3 to 7.2 down to 7 and later to 6.5 in more advanced stages of cancer and in metastases the pH drops to 6.0 and even down to 5.7 or lower. Our bodies simply cannot fight disease if our body pH is not properly balanced.

Clinically speaking, the gold standard for measuring a person's overall acid/base balance is blood pH. Blood pH is an overall composite of what is going on in the whole body and is regulated primarily by your kidneys, lungs, intestines, and liver. To know exactly what is going on at the cellular level would be ideal, but it is not clinically practical to measure the pH within the cell. Practically, the most useful pH measure for following one's diet and consumption of acid-producing or alkalising foods is to measure the urine pH.

Urine pH values:

In a pH balanced body. Urine is slightly acid in the morning, (pH = 6.5-7.0) generally becoming more alkaline (pH = 7.5-8.0) by evening in healthy people primarily because no food or beverages are consumed while sleeping. Whereas, during the day the body buffers the pH of the food and beverages consumed by releasing electrolytes and the pH level goes up. This process allows the kidneys to slowly begin the elimination process.

Outside the range implies that cells are being burdened with caustic pH fluids within and without surroundings. Long-term experience outside this range is unhealthy. However, the pH of urine can range from an extremely unhealthy low of 4.5 to a high of 8.5, which it tolerates a little easier, depending on the acid/base status of the extracellular fluids. A high pH value may indicate the body is over buffering to compensate for a physiological system that is too acidic.

Range of Urine pH Values

UNHEALTHY: pH < 6.0 NEUTRAL (Healthy): pH = 6.5 to 8.0.

Generally, when urine pH is 6.0 and below for extended periods of time, it is an indication that the body's fluids elsewhere are too acid, and it is working overtime to rid itself of an acid medium. Thus, when urine pH is normal, then the blood pH is normal, but when the urine pH is overly acid, the body releases too many electrolytes to keep the pH level normal and maintain life. Easy-to-take urine buffer test strips are available to indirectly determine the safety of all body fluids, including blood.

Urine pH can change quickly and by large amounts (2-3 pH units) in response to a person's diet. Thereby, urine pH provides you with rapid feedback regarding the nature of your diet. A rapid change in urine pH does not signify that a rapid change in blood pH will follow. However, if urine pH is constantly measured as acidic over long periods of time (months), it is indicative that the body is chronically producing large amounts of acid (most likely from acid-generating foods). If your urine pH is constantly measured as alkaline over time, this is an indicator that your diet is overall net-alkalising, and your body is not likely to be acidic.

Urinary pH Test: The pH of the urine indicates how the body is working to maintain the proper pH of the blood. The urine reveals the alkaline building (anabolic) and acid tearing down (catabolic) cycles. The pH of urine indicates the efforts of the body via the kidneys, adrenals, lungs and gonads to regulate pH through the buffer salts and hormones. Urine can provide a fairly accurate picture of body chemistry, because the kidneys filter out the buffer salts of pH regulation and provide values based on what the body is eliminating. Urine pH can vary from around 4.5 to 9.0 for its extremes, but the ideal range is 6.5 to 7.2.

17

Outside of Conventional Medicine

> *It is difficult to get a medical practitioner to understand, as well as agree with something, when his professional standing is dependent upon his not understanding or agreeing with it!*

The term "complementary and alternative treatments" covers many diverse forms of treatment. Complementary and alternative therapies are a broad range of treatments that are outside of conventional medicine and are used to treat or prevent illness and promote health and well-being. Practitioners of complementary therapies are not trained to diagnose disease. The area of complementary and alternative medicine is controversial and changes regularly. Therapies that are considered "complementary" or "alternative" in one country may be considered conventional in another. Therapies that are currently considered alternative may become more mainstream over time, as researchers discover their effectiveness and they become integrated into mainstream health care practice.

Both complementary and alternative medicines include many different healing approaches that people use to prevent illness, reduce stress, prevent or reduce side effects and symptoms, or control or cure disease. An approach is generally called complementary when it is used in addition to treatments prescribed by a doctor. An approach is often called alternative when it is used instead of treatments prescribed by a doctor. Research has shown that more than half of the people with cancer use one or more of these non-orthodox approaches.

Some common approaches include: visualisation or relaxation; acupressure and massage; homeopathy; vitamins or herbal products; special diets; psychotherapy; spiritual practices; energy healing, and acupuncture. After cancer treatment, many survivors want to find ways to reduce the chances of their cancer returning. Some worry that the junk foods they eat, over-stress in their lives, or their exposure to chemicals can put them at risk. You can be sure that junk food will cause problems! Cancer survivors also find that this is a time when they take a good look at how they take care of themselves and their health. This is an important start to living a healthy life after cancer. Also remember that stress can become a killer!

Complementary and alternative treatments can be used instead of conventional medicine, provided you have thoroughly researched the subject matter. There are some unscrupulous people out there! Forewarned is forearmed! However, if you decide to use complementary or alternative treatments it is important that you continue to see your doctor and keep him/her informed of the treatments you are having or considering. However, don't expect the doctor to agree with you for all your suggested treatments! Doctors are not trained to blindly accept unproven methods, no matter how successful they may appear.

Although most complementary and alternative treatments have a good safety profile, they are not 100 per cent proficient and there are serious safety concerns about some treatments. For example, some herbal preparations may interact harmfully with conventional drugs. It is therefore very important that your doctor knows exactly what you are taking or proposing to take.

Don't be nervous about telling your doctor what you are using—awareness of complementary and alternative treatment is increasing among the medical profession, and some doctors are sympathetic to its use. How widespread are complementary and alternative treatments?

At least one-in-four people are thought to have used complementary or alternative treatments in the past. In recent surveys, 85 per cent of medical students, 76 per cent of General Practitioners and 69 per cent of hospital doctors have said they feel that complementary treatments should be made available on the English National health service. This wide-spread interest helps to encourage research in the area.

One common concern is the difficulty in regulating such a varied range of treatments. Most forms of complementary and alternative treatments have one or more governing bodies, which set standards for the training and services provided and codes of conduct for practitioners. However, these are often self-regulated and membership tends to be voluntary. A report by the English House of Lords called for more regulation, and research to investigate effectiveness and safety. However, current regulation is still on-going.

Within Australia, complementary and alternative treatments are growing in numbers by interested people, many of whom are not convinced that orthodox medicine has all of the answers for all forms of cancer. There is still hope out there!

18

Controversy Between Various Treatments

Smart patients in the United States of America understand the controversy before they make treatment choices!

If you're thinking of trying alternative treatments, complementary and/or integrative medicines, there might be a treatment you've heard of and want to try. Or you may have exhausted the conventional route and would like to know what can be done using alternative medicine. Or maybe you just want to be stay healthy and are interested in finding out new methods to help you. Whatever your personal situation, you undoubtedly have many questions to ask.

Can alternative medicine actually help you? Are you covered by insurance for any of these treatments? Are there any treatments that you should steer clear of? Protect yourself with the information you need to make a smart decision about alternative care.

Few controversies exist in modern medicine like those stirred up by complementary and alternative medicine (CAM). While some doctors and patients embrace them and make use of CAM, even integrating them with conventional treatments, other professionals and patients dispute their effectiveness, believing that they may be dangerous, and even think they are either a joke, or a criminal activity. The fact is, the truth depends on which aspect of CAM is being discussed.

One of the biggest differences between CAM and conventional medicine, and the basis to much of the controversy, is the evidence, or lack thereof, that CAM actually works to improve a patient's well-being. Most conventional medicine aims at making recommendations to patients that are grounded in evidence accumulated through clinical trials and other research. The majority of this research has been performed on conventional treatments, such as pharmaceutical drugs. Little evidence proves alternative or complementary treatments actually work. But that is not necessarily because those treatments do not work! It is that most have not been researched thoroughly or at all! Why the discrepancy in the amount of research between the two approaches? Let me be frank! It comes down to one word—profit.

Most research is supported by for-profit organisations like pharmaceutical and medical device manufacturers to prove that their drug or device really works. With proof, they can get Federal Department of Agriculture approval to sell their drug or device. Even research being done in non-profit organisations such as universities and academic medical centres is mostly being conducted through grants and foundations developed by for-profit companies. There isn't as much money to be made if the evidence for CAM treatments is shown to exist. Further, no research needs to be done to achieve FDA approval (see below.) Therefore, except for government research projects through the National Centre for Complementary and Alternative Therapy (part of the National Institutes of Health), the research simply does not exist.

If the research doesn't exist, then effectiveness of CAM treatments can't be proved one way or the other. Maybe it works. Maybe it doesn't. We just don't know. That means we mostly rely on anecdotal evidence. For some integrative medical professionals, and patients, anecdotal evidence is all that's required to decide a CAM treatment is useful. There are no studies to prove that the pulp of an aloe vera plant can provide burn relief, yet many of us grow aloe vera plants for just that purpose! Natural supplements are a multi-billion dollar business in the United States, yet most of those supplements have no proof to show they work. Some even have proof that shows they don't! Nevertheless, people still buy them. Sceptics will tell you that spending money on CAM supplements and treatments are a complete waste of money. It may even be dangerous.

Choosing a CAM treatment may cause a conflict with a current, conventional treatment, which can result in additional medical problems when they are used together. Using a CAM treatment in place of a conventional treatment may mean improvement in health, or, it may mean death! However, even these reports are anecdotal. The evidence of the conflicts and deaths is not based on studies or clinical trials either.

One other caution about anecdotal evidence: It is the basis for quackery—the illegal and dangerous practice of selling treatments to sick, debilitated and dying patients who spend their money on products and procedures that don't work, because they are desperately looking for a cure, and hopeful that anything at all will help them. In particular, the Internet is rife with quacks trying to sell their useless, expensive and, sometimes, dangerous products and treatments to these people.

Anecdotal evidence is not nearly enough for many conventional medical doctors. And that raises another problem, and controversy—honesty. And, sometimes, a patient makes a choice on a simple belief, based on no more than something someone else has told them, or a label they have read on a bottle of supplements, or reading a website that may, or may not, be credible. Then, they decide their doctor might be upset or pass judgment on them for taking that supplement or choosing that treatment. Therefore, they don't tell the doctor. Withholding such information can be very dangerous.

For example, a patient might believe that taking a certain supplement will relieve their pain, or boost their immunity. In fact, it may conflict with a drug the doctor prescribed, or it may simply negate the benefit of the drug (or vice versa.) An example of this is the use of drugs for gastro-reflux disease (GERD), called proton pump inhibitors (like Prilosec, Nexium,

Previcid, Aciphex and others), combined with some forms of calcium supplements taken to strengthen bones and teeth. The drug cancels out the benefits of the calcium. The wiser patient is honest with his or her doctor.

Another major problem for patients and doctors who want to choose a CAM treatment, is that most have not gone through any form of approval process with the FDA. Conventional treatments are rigorously tested, and must apply to the FDA in order to be released and marketed to the public. CAM treatments do not require FDA approval.

Since CAM therapies do not have that same requirement, it's difficult to judge whether they are safe or not. There is also the question about using the word "natural." Many herbal supplements, for example, claim to be natural. However, natural and safe, are not necessarily the same thing! Arsenic is natural and deadly. So is hemlock, among many other toxic plants.

A wise patient will learn more about how these studies work and the controversies behind gathering the evidence. One of the important aspects of choosing the right doctor is to check into his or her qualifications. Medical education, state licencing, and board certification—these are very important credentials that improve the chances you will receive the advice and follow through you need. There are formal educational opportunities, including degrees and certificates, for some (but not all) CAM approaches. There is formal training for chiropractic, massage treatment, and doctors of naturopathy, for example. Please note, a naturopath and a doctor of naturopathy are not the same, especially outside of America.

The people who practice CAM medicine may or may not need to be educated or licensed. Some are. Some aren't. With few exceptions (and those exceptions vary from state to state) anyone may read a book, take a course, or simply hang out a sign saying they are a practitioner of whatever treatment they claim. To find out whether your particular treatment choice requires a license in your state, you can do a search for the name of the treatment, your state and license. Example: "acupuncture, Texas, license." If you learn the treatment requires a license, then be sure the practitioner you choose is licensed.

Before you make alternative or complementary medicine choices, be sure to understand the following:

- What are Alternative, Complementary and Integrative Medical Therapies?
- Finding Credible, Reliable and Objective Health Information on the Internet.
- How to Talk to Your Doctor About Alternative and Complementary Medicine.
- Healthcare Fraud—Quacks, Snake Oil and False Advertising.

WHAT DO U.S. PHYSICIANS THINK ABOUT ALTERNATIVE TREATMENTS?

A survey of 276 Colorado physicians was published in the May 2002 issue of Archives of Internal Medicine. Physicians were asked about their attitudes toward alternative medicine and their pattern of recommendation and personal use. Here are the interesting findings:

At the doctor's office, patients are sometimes asked about their use of alternative therapies.

- 8% always ask about alternative therapy use.
- 23% asked their patients about alternative treatment use more than half of the time.
- 52% asked about alternative treatment use less than half of the time 17% never ask.
- Many doctors do not feel comfortable discussing alternative therapies with their patients.
- 9% had a very positive attitude toward discussing alternative therapies with patients.
- 35% had a somewhat positive attitude.
- 40% were neutral.

- 14% had a somewhat negative attitude.
- 2% had a very negative attitude.

Patients want information from their doctors about the safety and effectiveness of alternative treatments. In this study, 59% of the doctors had been asked about alternative treatments. Patients requested information about:

- Acupuncture (59%).
- Herbal (botanical) medicine (55%).
- Chiropractic (52%).
- Alternative treatment in general (49%).
- Massage treatment (41%).
- Special diet (35%).
- Megavitamins (32%).
- Biofeedback (29%).
- Relaxation (28%).
- Homeopathy (21%).
- Folk Medicine (17%).
- Yoga (16%).
- Hypnosis (14%).

Nearly half (48%) of the doctors surveyed had recommended alternative medicine to a patient. Interestingly, 24% of the doctors had personally used alternative medicine, and this was strongly associated with the likelihood of recommending alternative medicine to patients. Some of the treatments, doctors personally used were: massage therapy (24%), relaxation techniques (17%), alternative medicine in general (16%), herbal treatment (14%), yoga (11%), and acupuncture (10%).

Doctors are interested in learning more about alternative medicine to address patient concerns. In this survey, 60% of doctors wanted to learn more, 24% said they were unsure or maybe wanted to learn more, and 16% said they did not want to learn more. The doctors recommended these therapies to their patients:

- Massage therapy (48%).
- Relaxation techniques (41%).
- Acupuncture (35%).
- Biofeedback (35%).
- Chiropractic (30%).
- Alternative medicine in general (28%).
- Herbal medicine (21%).
- Yoga (16%).
- Hypnosis (15%).

Note: Surveys were delivered to 705 physicians. Of these, 302 (43%) were returned. This must be considered when interpreting the survey results because they may not accurately reflect the physician population.

19
Cancer "Cures"

It is all very well to speak about cancer treatments, but the majority of cancer sufferers and others, really want to know is whether the treatment is pain free and if the treatment is a one-off success story or life extending.

The treatment that I used, with a few variations, has allowed Vernon Johnston to be cancer free for about five years. As for myself I am approaching nearly four years free of melanoma pain and any signs of lumps, and I feel as if I shall continue in this manner for some time to come. You know how you feel without having to have a doctor confirm it! But, what does going into remission, and the cancer being benign actually mean?

Here is one definition of remission: A period during which symptoms of disease are reduced (partial remission) or disappear (complete remission). With regard to cancer, remission means there is no sign of it on scans or when the doctor examines you. Doctors use the word "remission" instead of cure when talking about cancer because they cannot be sure that there are no cancer cells at all in the body. The cancer could come back in the future, although there is no sign of it at the present.

Complete remission means: the disappearance of all disease for longer than one month.

The tumour-free time period, is dated from the very first, not the last, therapy session. Patients with tumours that recur within one month of treatment ending are considered to have had no remission. Disappearance of all disease is complete remission; reduction tumour size by more than 50 per cent is considered partial remission.

A newly diagnosed cancer patient has several options to deal with their cancer:

- Have surgery, chemotherapy and radiation (i.e. orthodox treatments), as prescribed by their doctor (this may include orthodox treatments other than surgery, chemotherapy and radiation).
- Have surgery, chemotherapy and radiation, but drop out of the treatment program prematurely.
- Refuse all treatments (i.e. have zero surgery, zero chemotherapy, zero radiation, zero alternative treatments, etc.).
- Have alternative treatments after extensive orthodox treatments and after doctors have given up all hope for the treatment of this patient.
- Have alternative treatments after some orthodox treatments, but the patient dropped out of the orthodox treatment program prematurely.
- Have alternative treatments instead of orthodox treatments (i.e. they refused orthodox treatments).

Note that in the last three items, which deal with alternative treatments, there are over 400 different alternative cancer treatments, thus there are really over 400 options available to a newly-diagnosed cancer patient. Therefore, the most important point to be dealt with is: how does any patient determine which treatment plan is best for them? We all have our own choices! I took mine and was more than happy with the results!

IS THE CURE RATE FOR ORTHODOX MEDICINE CORRECT?

In its cancer statistics, the American Cancer Society (ACS) listed some of their cancer cure rates as high as 45%-55%. Yet, the general public are discovering through reading, and other sources, that the true rate for orthodox cancer treatment is less than 3%!

Who is telling the truth? Answer: The reason why the ACS and other cancer societies' claim such high figures is due to the fact that they use a "five-year survival" rate, i.e., ability to live for five years.

This is an arbitrary figure and there is no scientific basis for choosing this particular number. That means if the cancer originates at the liver, and after five years, you have no liver cancer, but you have developed lung cancer, you are still considered cured and your figure is added to the cure rate! Or, you have cancer and you survived for five years, but you died from their cancer treatment after five years and one day, you are still considered cured, according to their cure rate statistics. Or, you have been "cured" of cancer by orthodox treatment and due to the destruction of your immune system caused by the toxic treatment, you fall sick by catching a simple cold or pneumonia and you died. You are still considered "cured" of cancer, and your name is added to the cure rate.

This is totally unacceptable and a manipulation of cancer statistics to deceive the general public. Natural treatments have thirty times higher cure rate than orthodox treatments of radiation therapy, chemotherapy and surgery.

Source: Cancer-treatment-Tips.com.

20

Recovery From Loss of Hope

Hope is a word that is used often in our culture, a concept that is promoted by some and disparaged by others. Yet, hope is not wishful thinking!

When I heard the doctor say that I had up to six months to live, I felt I was a dead man walking. It was not the feeling an employee feels when he is certain he is to be fired in the near future. Nevertheless, having faced death's door on three occasions, I felt as if I had nothing of true value, no heart, no mind of my own. In a nutshell, I was temporarily suffering from loss of hope.

Even now, my heart often races every time I visit my doctor, a man, who is of the firm opinion that orthodox medicine is the only answer to eradicating cancer. I cannot help the feeling that the visit will rest on a biased diagnosis and I'll be back in hospital sooner than I need to be. Indeed, I was suffering from loss of hope! Where is the hope in a visitation to such a doctor?

Recovering from a loss of hope is a process which does not happen overnight! I think what is needed to sustain such a condition during such times is a source of love that can be consistently present with such sufferers through the turbulent ups and downs of emotion that are being experienced. All of us human beings are imperfect, and it may be that our friends, family members or counsellors are not always able to hold a consistent presence of love for sufferers during these difficult times. Therefore, the answer appeared to be, for me, at least, to keep on trusting in hope, for hope is certainly full of love, if we can only recognise this fact.

On the other side of the issue, sufferers with stage II cancer have been found to have had significantly higher levels of hope than those with stage IV cancer—the last stage for cancer. The presence of physical symptoms and pain may have an influence on a sufferer's degree of hopelessness. Therefore, it seems that it all depends on a person's attitude toward their cancer and themselves. Some see cancer as a death sentence, while others regard cancer as a learning curve, where the degree of pain is judged on a day-to-day or even an hour-by-hour basis, pondering on the lessons to be learned from this disease. Some people resort to prayer with its comforting effects, while others feel resigned to their fate. But hope is the main ingredient that allows people to encourage their sagging strength and low mind set, thus giving a boost, even if is only a slight boost, to the immune system. For the immune system has been weakened by the effects of cancer. I cannot stress enough about the benefits of having everlasting hope!

One point that is not recognised nearly enough is the spirit of the actual cancer sufferer. Yet, the most important part is often overlooked. That is giving little credence to the value of hope! I would strongly suggest to never, never, ever give up on your hold of hope! Because without hope a patient can all too soon become lost in a mind full of confusion that quickly turns to despair.

Yes! People can recover from loss of hope! Counting your blessings may be one point that you may have missed. A visit to any hospital will soon show how lucky you are, when there are many people far worse off than yourself. Hope has a marvellous recovery rate and all you need to do is to keep on hoping!

It is easy enough to over simplify, but we all have been informed in one way or another that excessive stress, anxiety and fear in our lives do cause real health problems. Anti-depression and anti-anxiety drugs are supposed to help cancer sufferers cope with their over-stressed lives. But, it is not enough! There has to be another way. And there is, by having a strong belief in hope! Yet, it is all confusing and difficult being a cancer sufferer wanting a new drug or treatment to be available and one that doesn't take a further twelve years to develop. However, once people accept that they have cancer, they often feel a sense of hope. There are many reasons to feel hopeful.

An alternative cancer treatment can be successful and thousands of people who have had cancer are alive today as a result of alternative treatments. It has to be said that many doctors ponder on the chances that hope may or may not help your body deal with cancer. Their professional training does not allow them to have an open mind and, therefore, positive attitude and feelings of hope are considered to be hallucinatory and, even though scientists are looking at the question of whether a hopeful outlook and positive attitude really helps people feel better, the main body of the medical profession thinks otherwise. Nevertheless, here are some ways the cancer sufferers can build their sense of hope:

1. Look for reasons to hope; believe in hope!
2. You may find hope in nature, or your religious or spiritual beliefs. Or, you may find hope in stories about people with cancer who are leading active lives once again, through taking alternative treatments.

Hope is a word that is often used in our culture, a concept that is supported by some and disparaged by others. Yet, hope is not simply wishful thinking! There are no guarantees in life and that is where hope invigorates people enough to face another minute, another hour, and yes, another day and with it, comes a smile of realisation that hope is true to you as well as me! Hope brought me through my trauma and it can for other cancer sufferers, too! All because hope builds on one's confidence that you can . . . and will, survive!

21

How a Cancer Diagnosis Can Affect a Spouse

A cancer diagnosis can also affect one's spouse more than one realises. Sometimes, the complex feelings and lifestyle changes caused by the diagnosis, its treatment, whether orthodox treatment or alternative treatment, or even trying to decide which treatment is even best to follow. In a word, it can become overwhelming for everyone. Understanding the potential changes in the way you relate to your spouse, in the way they relate to you, may help you take steps to foster a healthy, mutually supportive relationship during this extremely challenging period in your life. Cancer has the greatest effect on marriages and other long-term partnerships. After a diagnosis of cancer, both partners may experience sadness, anxiety, anger, hopelessness and fear. A fear that being a caregiver may disrupt their own future plans, such as following a particular career that is now suspect of even getting off the ground with the intended career vanishing before their very eyes.

There may be shifts in relationships and in the way spouses organise to take care of household chores or family activities. For some couples facing the challenges of cancer together strengthens their relationship and commitment. For others, especially those who struggled before the diagnosis, the stress of cancer may create ever more challenges. Although the effects of cancer vary from couple to couple, here are some changes that occur frequently in relationships.

Roles: Cancer may change you and your spouse's roles, and very often, in several unexpected ways. Some spouses become over-protective or controlling. This tendency may also affect the exchange of information both at home and with a Palliative Care team. Although it may seem normal or even generous to try to spare your spouse some details of the diagnosis or treatment, keeping secrets is not the answer. Being completely honest with each other is tantamount to the caring and sharing part of any marriage. It is of no benefit to either party to isolate each other from one another and the truth! Adjusting to a shift in roles does not come easily. A person who has always been in charge or served in those roles before, may struggle to take charge and provide care and, even more important, understanding!

These role changes often affect one's self esteem. Either partner may feel frustrated by the other's over-protectiveness or feel isolated when decisions aren't discussed openly. It is important to communicate with your spouse or partner, about your feelings and work together as best you can to make decisions about treatment, care giving, and other issues. It may help you to think about it as teamwork and plan your strategy together. With pen and paper, jot down what tasks or chores need to be done and negotiate who should assume primary responsibility for each. Learn more about how to communicate with your spouse about the cancer. Both the cancer suffer and the spouse may benefit from discussing whether or not to switch domestic chores or other jobs. In addition, although it may be challenging for both, it is important to readily accept outside help from friends, family members or professionals. Communicating openly about limitations and brainstorming possible solutions will help both feel more comfortable with changes in responsibilities. Because the physical and emotional needs often change frequently, as couples cope with cancer, it is important for both to communicate their special needs. Asking for help with basic activities of daily life, such as getting dressed or washing your hair, may be difficult. At the same time, you cannot assume that your spouse may even know or guess that you need help, or simply may not want to offend you by offering that help. Once again, it is tantamount to communicate openly and clearly express your needs to avoid the frustration and anger that can result from misinterpreting your spouse's behaviour.

Never forget! Both partners need extra reassurance that they are still very much loved. Cancer does drastically change the hopes and dreams that couples share. Plans for retirement, travelling, or even parenthood can change, causing feelings of sadness, anger and even fear of the unknown! The process of working together to meet new, short-term goals, such as finishing cancer treatment, can help couples feel more connected. For some, re-evaluating priorities may result in a better outlook on life. Things that seemed important before the cancer diagnosis may give way to new priorities, such as enjoying more time together.

The effects of cancer on your relationships with friends and family members vary widely, largely dependent on the close-ness of the relationship. Putting some goals on hold rather than abandoning them completely, sometimes helps, but not always. It is helpful to remember how your family reacts in a crisis and how you have all dealt with other difficult challenges and then plan your strategy for communicating news and asking for support. Many people do not know how to react to speaking to someone with cancer. Perhaps, it is a reminder of a fear of their future death. Who really knows? They just cannot face this issue.

However, your friends and family members will likely want to help you, but they might not know what you need or how to ask you. Be specific, direct and explicit about your needs and try not to make any assumptions about who will help and who will not. For example, ask friends and family to do your laundry, exercise the dog, or keep others up to date on your progress. But, if you find you have a well-meaning, but overbearing family member, who is complicating your efforts, then you, or some close family member will need to set limits. This may prove difficult, but it is best to be direct and let them know exactly what you need and can tolerate. One way to approach this is to say: "I appreciate your involvement, but your being here every day is making me tired. I think it best if you only come on Tuesday and Thursday next week and, maybe alternate other days the following week. Does that work for you?"

Try, as much as possible to keep in social contact with friends and family. Your friends might assume that you don't want to be invited to social events, therefore, let them know to keep inviting you, if that is your need. Meanwhile, let people know about your physical limitations; don't be afraid to cancel a date if you are physically or emotionally tired. People might not fully understand about how you feel or even themselves, but give them time to sort things out for themselves. But, always remember, they might not fully understand, after all.

Keep positive thoughts uppermost in your mind at all times, because your energy levels will appreciate your efforts!

22

Appreciation of My Devoted Caregiver

How does one really thank someone special for saving their life? Through gratitude, appreciation, or hold them in high esteem? As for me, I should like to use all of those terms interpreted by all of these words. Yet, a simple "thank you" does not ever seem enough. To my wife, Jeannie, please accept my deep appreciation for all of your efforts in helping me fight this metastacised melanoma cancer. We both know the many hours of stress that you endured all too well!

Therefore, as an example of Jeannie's devoted care to me, allow me to explain some of the trauma that a caregiver undergoes.

Caregivers of cancer patients are essential for ensuring the treatment of whatever type, orthodox or alternative treatment; continuity of care, social support and assisting the Palliative Care team and Social Worker within the system in achieving the patient's treatment goals. It is stated that 71% of women are the prime caregivers in Australia, and care giving can negatively impact on the caregiver's own health, well-being, immune system, risk of disease, e.g., heart disease and metabolic syndrome (high blood pressure), especially, when compared with non-caregivers.

It is all too easy to forget that the following passages are completely true, which involve Jeannie and myself, and reveals our experience of undergoing the day-to-day trauma of cancer. But what good is experience unless it is shared so that others, too, may learn certain lessons. I only hope that my readers will try to understand and comprehend the degrees of trauma that some caregivers and their particular cancer sufferers undergo. Some traumas are such that they can be filled with heart-wrenching stress, which, if not completely controlled end up as killers, not only in the literal sense but also as killers of that inner spirit that dwells in each and every one of us.

Being a caregiver for a cancer patient takes a special type of person. For example, Jeannie was such a person and one, who I might add, had had a full-time experience of looking after a previous husband for twenty-two long years. She never knew if he would ever recover from his debilitating disease. However, he eventually passed away without having the opportunity of expressing any gratitude to Jeannie for her never faulting duty of care.

Some months later, and for the first time in her life, Jeannie had the opportunity to do something that she had always dreamed of—to take up painting, but not the classic style of painting. Jeannie desired to become an abstract artist, and to this end, she attended an American college where she gained her Bachelor of Arts degree.

In the meantime, I cared for my first wife, Moira, for five years before she passed away. She had a leaking mitral valve condition whereby the liver consumed the blood and increased in size, extending into other organs. It was a sad situation, which extended over several years of illness and, finally, Moira passed away.

I was encouraged to go on the Internet to try to find a companion by my family. That was how I met Jeannie, an American, from California! We e-mailed each other for several months and during that time we discovered that we had more in common that we first imagined. We were both elated.

I invited Jeannie to visit me on the Gold Coast, in Queensland, to meet my family and to familiarise herself with Australian customs and mannerisms. She agreed and was delighted at the invitation. We got on extremely well. After a month I asked Jeannie to return to the States to talk things over with her family. After Jeannie's return to the States was when 9/11 erupted. We feared that we might not see one another again for several years as we expected war to break out. Therefore, we decided to get married in Hawaii in two months' time.

I fully realised by that stage that Jeannie was more than interested in abstract art and therefore, I arranged to take her to England, Scotland, and Paris, especially to see The Louvre, and the Musse d'Orsay Art Galleries. Then we flew to Florida to visit friends of mine and then flew to southern California to meet some of Jeannie's relatives and later flew to northern California to meet the remainder of her relatives. We all got on extremely well.

We flew home, where we discussed moving from the Gold Coast to a quiet lifestyle on Macleay Island, in the Morton Bay marine reserve, just off the coast of Queensland, near Redland Bay. We were content and happy for seven years. Then Jeannie received word that her eldest daughter Judy Laura, had cancer. We flew back to California to assist in driving Judy Laura for chemotherapy treatment, among assisting the family in other ways; this included travelling along six-lane highways crammed with traffic all doing about 75 miles per hour. After three months my visa expired and we had to leave America. It was a very sad occasion. Three months later Jeannie heard that Judy Laura was near to death. Unfortunately, as Jeannie's aircraft landed in Los Angeles, Judy Laura passed away. Jeannie remained on for the funeral and then came home well after Christmas.

That was when the trouble began—I contracted melanoma cancer!

Here are a few important issues to remember if and when you become a caregiver for someone with cancer.

When the person you care for is having treatment, life may seem less predictable. You may have to put some plans on hold because you are not sure what is ahead. Caregivers often find this uncertainty stressful. You may find it easier to cope if you focus on things you can control.

You may be able to schedule doctors' visits so you can attend with the person you're caring for. It may also help to learn more about cancer and possible treatment options, so you feel like you have more knowledge about what is happening.

Talking with family and friends about how you feel about caring, particularly if you are feeling angry (venting) may help you deal with these emotions.

You may feel uncomfortable talking to the person with cancer because you think they have a lot to deal with already and you are meant to be their support. It's understandable if you don't want to talk to the person with cancer, but try not to hold in all your feelings. You can share your feelings with friends or family members, or join a support group for caregivers

Organise your time! It may not be possible to do everything you want to do. You will need to manage your time.

- Prioritise your weekly tasks and activities.
- Use a personal planner/diary to keep track of information and appointments.
- Ask for help from family, friends or support services. For instance, someone might be able to make dinner or drive the person with cancer to treatment. Asking for help is not a sign of failure and it may relieve some pressure.
- Concentrate on one task at a time, e.g. making dinner.
- Avoid multiple shopping trips, e.g. do one large shop rather than going daily.

Looking after someone with cancer is not always easy or satisfying. Many caregivers say they feel over-burdened and resentful. However, many of them say focusing on the value they were adding through home caring helped them to cope and made them feel better.

Some of the rewards of caring include:

- learning new skills.
- strengthening your relationship as you demonstrate your love and commitment.
- satisfaction from helping someone in need.

::

During my radiation treatment an error occurred, whereby the radiation melted the myelin sheathing of the nerves in my neck, exposing the nerves. There was no medical solution, except permanent pain killers. The pain was so bad one night that I was advised to apply a heated wheat bag to the area to help soothe the pain. At the time I was taking a sleeping pill and during the night the wheat bag burned my skin until the skin was black. Next morning Jeannie attempted to swab the weeping blood, being careful of the pieces of flesh loosely hanging there. Jeannie continued to attend to this burn over the weekend, but by then she realised that the wound needed more expert advice and attention. We all have our limits of stress that we can withstand. Jeannie readily admitted to me that this wound was now beyond her capabilities and therefore, we called on the assistance of the Blue Care Organisation.

The Blue Care nurse, who happened to be male, arrived at our home and immediately recognised that the degree of my burn was extremely severe. The Blue Care nurse was actually amazed at Jeannie's courage and degree of competence at caring for this dreadful burn. Jeannie continued to attend to the other duties of assisting me, such as preparing our eighty per cent alkaline and twenty per cent acidic diet; checking I had taken the prescribed medication from the various drugs at the correct times; preparing fresh vegetables to be juiced each day; making appointments with medical professionals; attending to Department of Veterans' Affairs for special travel arrangements to travel to Brisbane to visit a specialist; and, driving me to and fro from the water transport on the island.

The melanoma cancer had metastacised, which was when I was told I had six months to live. I sought an alternative treatment and Jeannie spent time preparing the various herbs and special juices needed to help fight the cancer. As a result of this treatment, I perspired terrifically for two nights; I completely drenched my bed clothing as well as the bed. Then a catastrophe! I soiled the bed with several bouts of diarrohea. It was the toxins being expelled by my body and with it, dead cancer cells! But that was not the end of the matter. The alternative treatment went on for months. Then I contracted bowel cancer!

In a moment of deep stress and quite unbeknown to me, Jeannie asked our island doctor what exactly were my chances of survival from the bowel cancer. He replied: "At best, I would say a 30 per cent chance of survival!"

I can't imagine what went through Jeannie's head at that moment. It wouldn't have been pleasant.

In the meantime, I was in hospital and had had the bowel cancer operation via keyhole surgery. Later, I had two CT scans which caused a sensation among the oncologists, because the scans showed there was no signs of my former tumours and the two remaining spots were declared benign!

When told of this news, my mind went into a whirl! I had actually survived melanoma cancer in my shoulder/neck area, both lungs, my liver and melanoma bowel cancer! I wasn't the only one calling it a miracle. The oncologists were completely stunned by the scan results.

Then we received a phone call from America to say that Jeannie's second daughter, Jennie Flippen, had suddenly passed away. Both of Jeannie's daughters were only in their fifties. It was a mad rush to get Jeannie on an aircraft to America.

On her return to Australia, Jeannie's stress level was plainly observed by the Palliative Care team and even the Social Worker. They told her she needed a break from caring for me and when I returned from hospital it was arranged I go into respite care. During the week I was hospitalised, Jeannie phoned me every night saying she loved me and missed me. I returned the loving sentiments. On the Thursday I phoned Jeannie to inquire if she was all right and that I intended coming on the Friday. She agreed. When I returned, I noticed an immediate change in my wife. After embracing one another, Jeannie said:

"Frank, there's something I have to tell you. But first, would you like a cup of tea?"

I was taken aback slightly and murmured yes to a cup of tea. After which, Jeannie spoke in a firm tone:

"I have a girlfriend coming. But there's something I need to tell you . . . I can no longer care for you . . . I feel my abstract art career is far more important to me than my marriage!"

The girlfriend arrived and Jeannie left the house less than hour after I had returned home!

I looked around at the dining room and that was when I realised that all of her art work had been removed from the walls. On further investigation, I found that even her clothing had gone! Obviously, Jeannie had planned her move while I was in respite.

It was just before I went into hospital the last time that Jeannie confessed she had been to the doctor about my bowel cancer operation and what the doctor had said to her. It seemed the CT scans report had made no difference.

In Jeannie's mind she was overly concerned that the cancer would return, trapping her from her long-time dream of having an art career. Her past experience of looking after a previous husband for twenty-two years sprang to her mind and she just couldn't face another term of looking after me. This was her last opportunity to realise her dream of becoming an accomplished abstract artist.

She had made her plans methodically, although somewhat hurriedly as I was expected home within two days.

I was heartbroken and I cried a river. I just couldn't fully understand why! I needed what was lacking—honest communication about her level of stress, and a need to discuss everything fully. But I was denied any of this. I walked about in a daze for several hours and then phoned a friend. He decided that it best if my daughter arrived from the Gold Coast to stay with me.

Jeannie had previously phoned my son in Canberra to tell him that our marriage was over and that she would not be returning.

All of our friends and relations were completely shocked and distraught by Jeannie's completely out-of-character actions.

The rest has passed into history.

23

Reasons For Offering Genuine Hope

There is a growing knowledge in the belief that humans are more than just physical bodies. It is now strongly believed that humans are energetic beings. We can control our beliefs and our attitudes, and in doing so, focus on that, thereby strengthening our immune system, the natural healing mechanism within our bodies. That establishes an element of hope for sufferers of melanoma cancer. Helping the immune system fight cancer is tantamount to survival.

"You have cancer" are words that no one wants to hear. Yet, in Australia thousands of people will hear those words, and the impact on their lives and their families will be immense.

If there is good news, it's that there is a probability that several people diagnosed with cancer in Australia will survive their ordeal. The sad news, based on an article published online in the American Journal of Clinical Oncology, is that too many people will start their journey hearing those fateful words in a less than appropriate manner in a less than appropriate setting.

That is not only dismaying, it's appalling. And if physicians can't understand, empathise and even sympathise with their patients when physicians tell them their life is at risk, then physicians are in serious trouble as a profession.

In the United States of America, doctors have to inform patients of a cancer diagnosis. However, the physicians still have the problem regarding prognosis information[1]. In many cultures around the world, a cancer diagnosis is not routinely disclosed to patients[2].

A study was performed at the National Cancer Institute[3], where all of the 437 patients surveyed had been referred for treatment. The researchers asked them how they learned of their diagnosis, what the doctors told them at the time they received the news, where they were located when they had the conversation, and how long the conversation lasted.

The authors reported that a little over half the patients were told their diagnoses in their doctor's office, 18% over the phone, and 28% in the hospital. 44% of the conversations lasted less than 10 minutes, and 53% lasted more than 10 minutes. In about 31% of the conversations, no treatment plan was discussed. It is no surprise to anyone that patients were more satisfied with the experience—if you can say that you can be satisfied with hearing you have cancer—with discussions, other than by telephone, with longer time and with an explanation of treatment options.

It should be pointed out that this group of people was generally better educated, financially better off and a majority of patients had brain cancer, leukaemia and lymphoma.

When you delve deeper into the report, you find some interesting information. Here is where the article gets disheartening:

- Of the patients (28% of the group) who were in the hospital when they were told their diagnoses, 43% were told in their hospital room where maybe there was a semblance of privacy. But 23% were told in the emergency room, 13% in the recovery room, 7% in the radiology department and 13% in other locations in the hospital.
- 22% of the patients were told they had cancer by a medical oncologist, which means some other doctor(s) probably did all the diagnostic work but left the bad news to an oncologist. I suspect that many of the

patients guessed on their own they had cancer if another doctor had referred them to a cancer specialist for a consultation. To me, that seems a bit harsh. 4% of the patients were told by a non-physician, including radiology technicians, nurses, physician assistants and relatives.

- 39% of the patients were alone when told of their cancer diagnosis.
- 8% of the patients had a less than one minute conversation about their diagnoses.
- 36% said the conversation lasted between one and 10 minutes.
- 15% of the patients lost trust in their physician as a result of the conversation, based on poor communication and general dissatisfaction.
- Finally, there are the quotes in the article that really had me taking a moment to digest: "My doctor at the time called me on Valentine's day to say I had a lesion in my chest . . . he left this message on my home answering machine"; "The doctor telephoned and left a voice message saying you have lymphoma . . . call me if you have any questions"; "The neurologist called saying he had made arrangements (for me) to see a neuro-surgeon. I asked why? He replied, "You've got a brain tumour and hung up."

Maybe, I should look on the bright side of this report, and realise that the majority of patients were told their diagnoses with empathy and respect, in a reasonably private location and given sufficient time and attention. But the problem is that a significant minority of patients were not, and that is disturbing.

Years ago, it was customary for patients not to be told anything about their cancer diagnoses. The exception was for women with breast cancer, because it was difficult to ignore the situation when they woke up after surgery and saw that their breast was gone and their chest was covered in bandages. But for many others—no matter how obvious the situation—families and physicians conspired to keep them in the dark since there was so little that could be done.

An intern was sitting beside the bed of a man who was dying from lung cancer. He knew his diagnosis and that his days were limited, his family knew his diagnosis—but they demanded that the medical team not inform the patient of his circumstances. The charade may have been intact, but the emotions were not. That man said a great deal to me that night, and I still recall his distress at not having a final moment of openness and honesty with his family.

Times have changed, and patients and families are more empowered as a result. Patients are now routinely told of their diagnoses, and hopefully they and their families are active participants in their treatment decisions and knowledge of their disease. We clearly could do better in that regard, but we are making progress.

Obviously, most physicians care deeply about their patients. But the medical world is changing, just like everything else in our society. Patients are increasingly having difficulty establishing long term relationships with a primary care clinician, whether that be a physician or other health professional. Medical care is increasingly episodic as opposed to long term, and our care delivery is fragmented into specialties where too often there is no "captain of the ship."

Telling patients bad news is never easy, and although there are courses and programs to help physicians communicate better, the reality is that there is no measured practice standard that tells us whether or not physicians communicate effectively with their patients, especially when physicians deliver difficult news.

Let all patients hope that physicians have not come to a time when empathy and understanding don't count. Perhaps, patients should look at the brighter side of this report in that most doctors do it right. But the fact is that too many physicians do not.

If physicians are not able to tell people life-threatening news with some shred of sensitivity and dignity, then maybe some physicians are at risk of losing their human touch. That loss of humanity goes to the heart of what it means to be a doctor. And if the medical fraternity lose that, it would be tragic.

::

An Opposing View

An American physician took offense at the published findings of the National Cancer Institute's study and here is part of his comments:

"The best that Figg, *et al*, can propose to evaluate regarding the communication of a cancer diagnosis, are the patients' perceptions of the disclosure. It is important to comprehend that such perception means little without a corresponding understanding of how physicians actually communicate that information. Therefore, the survey can only claim to measure one side of patient-physician communication and only a limited portion at that. Although an important component of this communication, patients' perceptions do not inform the reader of physicians' energy, efforts, and investment in the effective and compassionate disclosure of a cancer diagnosis and consideration of an effective plan of care. Such a limited study tends only to confirm that a cancer diagnosis is a difficult topic of discussion and that patients' perceptions of that discussion can be the result of a single event. What Figg et al, seem to ignore is that this disclosure, this discussion, this ongoing relationship is a process—not an event."

References:

1. Kaplowitz SA, C ampo S, Chiu WT. "Cancer patients' desires for communication of prognosis information". Health Communication. 2002;14:221-41.
2. Holland JC, et al. "An international survey of physicians' attitudes and practices in regard to revealing the diagnosis of cancer." Cancer Invest. 1987;5:151-4.3.
    Figg WD, Smith EK, Price DK, et al. (2010) "Disclosing a Diagnosis of Cancer: Where and how does it occur?" J Clin Oncol 28:3630-3635.

24
An Orthodox Opinion

Over the many months I underwent surgical operations for the removal of seven cancer tumours, Dr. Chris Allen and I developed a special relationship, one of mutual trust and respect. After I received notification that I was clear of melanoma cancer I was elated, of course. Out of gratitude and respect for Dr. Allen I wrote to him updating my new situation.

I was rather surprised to receive a letter and I think it only fair that this and his opinion be expressed. Here, then is that letter:

14th December 2011
Dear Frank
Thank you for your lovely letter updating me on this remarkable turnaround in fortunes with the melanoma. I had heard from Greenslopes Hospital when you were admitted there with a melanoma deposit in the large bowel and clearly you have had a good outcome under Dr. Nic Lutton's care. It was remarkable to see that those multiple lung and liver metastases had disappeared and I sincerely hope it was due to the healthy approach you had taken to living and your diet. Frank you are now my second patient who has had what we would call a spontaneous resolution of metastatic melanoma and it is a well-recognised albeit rare pheno-menon with melanoma. The 'spontaneous' is obviously due to something and whilst we will never know, I have no problems with yourself or anyone claiming it to be the result of dietary changes or any other form of alternative treatment. The only

medical explanation I can give is that your immune system finally got the upper hand against the melanoma. Hopefully what you have done is responsible for gaining that upper hand. In any case it really is heartening and I am very pleased for your change in fortune. It does not sound as though you will need my attentions any further, but if so then please feel free to come back and see me or update me at any stage.

All the best,
Yours sincerely
Dr. Chris Allen, MBBS MPhil FRACS.

I did have the occasion to return to see Dr. Allen. I wanted an explanation of the term "insignificant" regarding two spots on my liver on one of the CT scans.

Dr. Allen looked up the details on his computer screen and eased my mind by stating:

"Frank, in laymen's terms, this means that those spots are now benign. So you have no worries. You have been most fortunate!"

::

Do I fear the recurrence of my melanoma cancer? It is common enough among most cancer survivors, and if, and when it comes to facing that situation, I shall probably be no different to anyone else. However, and it is a big however! I have my bicarbonate of soda and blackstrap molasses, my diagnostic strips and a mixture of my herbs at the ready! Also, I am ready to start blending my vegetables all over again. I am that confident!

The fear of recurring melanoma cancer may lead a person to over-interpret the significance of minor physical problems, such as a headache or joint stiffness. It is simply difficult to know what is "normal," and what needs to be reported to the doctor. Discussing the actual risk of cancer recurrence with your doctor and the symptoms to report can often reduce a person's anxiety. Maintaining your schedule of follow-up visits can also provide a sense of control. Although many cancer survivors describe feeling frightened and nervous at the time of routine follow-up visits, these feelings may ease with time. Whatever you do, do not panic! Retain your positive position throughout all trauma and, praying isn't a bad idea either!

During my cancer journey there were times when I was unsure whether I wanted to reveal to certain people that I had been diagnosed with stage IV melanoma cancer. One thing, I was certain—I did not want pity!

Being a cancer survivor means different things to different survivors. There is no right or wrong way to feel about sharing one's diagnosis or any information about your cancer journey. Whether or not one reveals their cancer journey is *their* choice and theirs alone!

There were several reasons why it was not easy for me to tell others that I was a cancer survivor, especially after surviving the tiger attack and being swept out to sea! Survivors all have their own personal reasons for not wanting to open up to certain people. I was unsure as to how people would react to such a remarkable finding that I was totally free of melanoma cancer! I felt like a freak in a circus show!

How did I react returning to my doctor to ask for a follow-up of my earlier CT scans, especially, when I knew he wasn't open-minded regarding alternative treatments? I figured that was his challenge! I had already faced my fears—and won!

::

On May 8, 2012, I received notice that my recent three CT scans, plus a bone scan, carried out at a Private Gold Coast Hospital, had proved that there was still no cancer in my body!

The CT scan report states:

Report date: 2/5/ 2012

Impression: On this occasion the hepatic lesion in the right lobe that was seen on prior scans appears to have almost completely resolved. There is a single tiny middle lobe. No other evidence of metastatic disease.
Dr. Shane Thompson.
Bone scan results:
No evidence of metastatic disease.
Dr. Shane Thompson.

This surely signifies that something very important has been proven through taking an alternative treatment! I figure that I can confidentially say . . . I rest my case!